Mental Health and Well-being

This book analyses mental health, well-being, and their interdependence from an Indian perspective. It offers critical insights on mastering wellness, stress, and coping; suffering and healing; and achieving work–life balance.

Describing key concepts of the Indian philosophical thought with contemporary implications, the volume focuses on explaining the how mental health and mental well-being are correlated. It examines the dynamic interplay of biological, social, psychological, ecological, cultural, religious, and spiritual factors that affect individuals in their everyday lives and act as contributing factors to their illness or wellness. The book also explores in-depth Indian traditions of spirituality and their significant contributions to mental well-being, including discussions on concepts found in Ayurveda and Yoga.

This book will be of interest to students, researchers, and teachers of psychology, applied psychology, clinical and counselling psychology, and wellness. It will also be very helpful for academicians, mental health professionals, counsellors, and those working in health and well-being industries.

Navin Kumar is a professor of psychology at the Bhim Rao Ambedkar College, Delhi University, India. With 25 years of teaching experience, he is the author of *Criminal Psychology*, published in 2015, and of *Media Psychology* and *Counselling Psychology,* both published in 2021. He is executive editor of *Academia*, an international multi-disciplinary biannual journal in social sciences, humanities, and languages.

He is a member of the Under-graduate and Post-graduate Board of Studies, Chaudhary Devi Lal University Sirsa, Haryana, and a member of the Board of Research Studies for Ph.D. Students at Amity University Noida, IILM University, Gurgaon, and Manav Rachna University, Faridabad. He has served as a member of M.Phil. Clinical Psychology Committee at IBHAS Dilshad Garden, Delhi. Dr Kumar has also been a member of UGC Learning Outcomes-based Curriculum Framework (LOCF) for Psychology, 2018, and a member of the Curriculum Committee, National Institute of Open Schooling (NIOS). He has conducted training workshops for Delhi Police, CRPF, NTPC, CISF, Power Grid and has previously been invited as a visiting faculty at National Law University, Delhi.

Dr Kumar has supervised 20 Ph.D. scholars as a guide/co-guide from Delhi University, Jamia Millia Islamia, and Amity University. He has presented several research papers, including a research paper at ICAP Paris, and has published more than 20 research articles in national and international journals. He has also completed several research projects with ICSSR, UGC, Delhi University, and Delhi Police and has been a coordinator for UGC and PG Pathshala for the subject Criminal Psychology (2017).

Mental Health and Well-being
An Indian Psychology Perspective

Navin Kumar

Routledge
Taylor & Francis Group
LONDON AND NEW YORK

First published 2023
by Routledge
4 Park Square, Milton Park, Abingdon, Oxon OX14 4RN

and by Routledge
605 Third Avenue, New York, NY 10158

Routledge is an imprint of the Taylor & Francis Group, an informa business

British Library Cataloguing-in-Publication Data
A catalogue record for this book is available from the British Library

ISBN: 978-1-032-02447-9 (hbk)
ISBN: 978-1-032-39633-0 (pbk)
ISBN: 978-1-003-35065-1 (ebk)

DOI: 10.4324/9781003350651

Typeset in Sabon
by Apex CoVantage, LLC

Contents

Preface

Nearly all problems faced by the world today require input from more than one discipline, and those individuals who participate in such problem-solving endeavours need to acquire and develop mindsets so that they are comfortable working in interdisciplinary settings. I have tried to follow the basic theme of this manuscript that explores the new, raises new questions, provides new answers, or ushers in or exemplifies new ways at thinking about the problem of mental health and well-being. It is worth mentioning that the problem of mental health and well-being has gained considerable currency among the academic and practitioners. The chapters in this book attempt to adopt a more practical approach and explore deeply the complexity of the mental health problems and help to bring out more sophisticated solutions. How do the theories of mental health experts relate to ordinary persons? Do they apply across the board – that is across diverse socio-cultural contexts? There are alternative theories and practices, disciplinary knowledge and understanding which can be relevant to acquire truly important perspectives on the notion of mental health and well-being.

This book is broad attempt to understand the well-being of modern man and the problems of the interaction between psychological, sociological, and technological factors. To understand the dynamic of the mental health and well-being, we must understand the fears, desires, passions, and reason of an individual in the contact of the culture which moulds him. In the thesis of this book, an individual freed from the bonds of traditional society has not got freedom in the positive sense of realization of his individual self. The modern capitalistic society has brought him independence, and rationality has made him alienated and thereby anxious and helpless. This book provides an analysis of unbearable alienation that an individual is confronted with in an industrial society which poses threats of new dependencies of work escaping from freedom.

In the modern capitalistic society, market regulates human relations. Being close to nature, work, and culture creates a system of being alone, and being together leads to deeper anxiety.

Modern man's selfishness has reached a remarkable degree, intending to master and control nature. But a close scrutiny presents no, it is contrary picture, and man has become estranged from this man-made world. The struggle for recognition and popularity in the modern society forces a man to be directed by others, creating a personality for oneself that is as mechanical as are products and services. Present scenarios of work and professionalism create a dependence of self-esteem on success.

The work–life balance is a relationship between employees and employer, which has assumed a spirit of manipulation functioning like a machine system. The divorce of the modern work ethic from its spiritual roots, led by the culture of consumption resulted into the production of stress at the workplace.

Tracing the novel features of causing stress, work–life balance, culture, spirituality, and suffering can contribute a role in the process of achieving mental health and well-being. The primary task of a book such as this is to present ideas that have been influential with regards to mental health and well-being. This book has seven chapters, and its primary focus is to discuss concepts like stress, work–life balance, culture, and spirituality from an Indian perspective; one of my concerns highlighted in this book is that only biomedical models cannot find solutions to mental health issues, and alternative approaches can also be explored. We live in a pluralist society in need of pluralism in all walks of life, including healthcare. Huge numbers of people are afflicted by chronic mental health problems whose symptoms can be non-organic or medically unexplained. There are numerous researches emphasizing on the link between poverty and mental health problems. Many alternative approaches like Ayurveda and yoga can be used to get rid of mental health problems. The process of suffering and healing is influenced by culture, attitude, beliefs, and spiritual orientation. Chapter 1 deals with fundamentals of mental health and well-being. It introduces the historical antecedents and details of mental health. I have tried to provide an introduction to the topics described in detail in the subsequent chapters. It also includes a discussion on the limitations of Western approaches. This chapter only presents a bird's-eye view of the field indicating a paradigm shift in the understanding of mental health.

Chapter 2 covers basic areas related to stress and coping. It also provides an overview of researches and approaches that are important in relation to mental health and well-being. Epigenetic mechanisms are implicated in the processes through which social stressors erode health in humans, while advances in technology have provided many benefits to society. New technology has also led to a substantial reduction in the amount of incidental physical activity. Relentless demands for increased profits and improved performance coupled with reduced resources predispose employees to stress and ill-health. Of all the concepts which have emerged to describe the effects of capitalism on the human world, most important is 'reification' which is a process by which men and women are turned into objects or things. In this period of capitalism and globalization, reification is best understood as a form of social and cultural anxiety. Digital stress concept examines and elucidates this effect of Internet-mediated communication based on perceived stress. Information and communication technology (ICT) has become an integral part of everyday life.

A large number of studies indicate the inherent risk of imposition of stress on Internet users. Fear of missing out, social pressure, and peer pressure result in higher level of communication overload. In the contemporary context of networked publics, relational exchanges are transacted in much more open environments resulting into digital stress. Chapter 2 provides a detailed description of psychological health effects and motivational origin of digital stress. This chapter will help its readers with a key to develop an awareness of how to interpret and react to circumstances and develop coping skills to manage stress. Chapter 3 is based on ecology and well-being principles and its human behaviour. This chapter reveals the psychological dimensions of environmental psychology. Behaviour is important for ecology because many ecological outcomes are the result of behavioural processes. There are strong relationships between attitudes towards the environment and ecological behaviour. Ecological knowledge is related to the role of the environment in human life, and this knowledge helps in shaping the attitude towards the environment. A growing amount of empirical evidence is revealing the value of natural experience for a good mental health.

Several aspects of contemporary living are associated with least contact with nature leading to mental health effects. Mental health and well-being may differ, being influenced by factors of economic status, residential location, personality traits, culture, and gender.

Indian approach towards environment has been discussed from the perspective of Vedas, Gita, Jainism, and Buddhism. It highlights a harmonious and reciprocal landing between man and his/her environment. The pattern of meaningful interaction with the environment can lead to higher levels of subjective well-being. Psychiatrists and other mental health professionals focus on an understanding of mental health from an environmental perspective. The context that the socio-ecological model provides helps us to consider the range of strategies available to promote mental well-being.

Chapter 4 is intended to be a contribution to the growing body of theoretical and empirical work in the area of workplace well-being. It encompasses the socio-cultural phenomena examining relations between work–life balance and well-being. For reasons to be more explored, I believe that work–life balance can provide a fundamental ground work for well-being that is scientifically rigorous. Our current notion of a healthy workplace has evolved over the years deriving from diverse disciplines of environment, health, and psychology. This chapter addresses that the contextual elements of a healthy workplace and the components surrounding positive psychology have been examined revealing the dynamics within the organization that influence employee flourishing and human resiliency. It also deals with the concept of occupational identity which describes the self-image association with one's profession. The socio-cultural factors play an important role regarding the choice and conceptions about a person's occupational identity. Indian concept of work as worship and Karma theory of action are quality additions in understanding workplace well-being.

The chapter 5 on culture and well-being prescribes a rich descriptive relationship between culture and work–life balance. There is a growing body of empirical research that highlights the role of organizational environment on work–life balance. The sensitivity to employee's family demands and co-operative attitude with co-workers may lead to positive outcomes. Work–life integration in today's unpredictable and fast-paced society is critical in the cultivation of a healthy work environment. Team-building exercises help to create supportive relationships. The concepts of consumption and its relationship with well-being have been presented in this chapter. Consumerism is a tendency for the pursuit of status and happiness through material possessions. Ample research shows that materialists are, on average, not the happiest people. Indian culture of well-being highlights the unique Indian traditions such as joint family system belief in Karma and Ahimsa (non-violence) with their implications on well-being. The chapter 6 on spirituality and well-being provides conceptual ideas to understand the relation between two. An attempt has been made to produce fascinating connections between religion, spirituality, and well-being. You will find selective focus on key ideas related to psychology, religion, and spirituality. Religion and psychology share a common concern with the quality of human existence. They hope to offer guidance to the people seeking a meaningful, fulfilling, and happy lives. There are some paradoxical aspects dealt with in this chapter. Examples include scientists insisting upon empirical evidence whereas spiritual theorists emphasizing eternal experiences beyond measurement. All of life something that is beyond us but also within us. The concepts of theism and rationality spirituality have been part and parcel of our day-to-day common language. Spirituality encompasses elements of inner awareness including a sense of mystery and mastery providing unity of oneself and others. The concepts of gratitude, hope, and forgiveness have important implications for well-being.

The last chapter 7 on suffering and healing provides an introduction to these concepts and that human suffering has biological, psychological, and existential aspects. The emotional, cognitive, and spiritual sufferings of human beings can't be separated from ecological, social, and political conditions. Suffering from the past for the sense of the meaning of life is a form of special form of emotional, cognitive, and spiritual suffering. People may suffer from a variety of harmful circumstances, and lacking any sense for same meaning in life is a fundamental form of emotional, cognitive, and spiritual suffering. Suffering and healing vary a lot according to suitable ways to finding meaningful ways even in crisis. According to Buddhist traditions, eightfold path to truth can relieve one from all sufferings of life. Buddhist spirituality is associated with the end of suffering through the enlightened knowledge of reality. One requires compassion, meditation, and wisdom to get relieved from sufferings. The paradise lies within ourselves, and only a conditioning of mind is required to experience bliss in the adverse situations. Within our own selves, there is a stillness and sanctuary to which you can retreat at any time and be yourself. Indian perspective considers *Dukha* (suffering) and *Sukha* (Happiness) as two sides of the same coin. It is our attitude towards life that makes us happy or unhappy. Isolation, anchoring, distraction, and sublimation are the ways to overcome suffering. Mindfulness meditation is a powerful mental training to calm both mind and body. Mindfulness meditation involve simple deep breathing techniques to free oneself from worries.

I have tried to set mental health and well-being in the larger socio-cultural context in which they operate. This textbook explains key concepts related to mental health and well-being, revealing diverse dimensions, and there is a lengthy discussion of the Indian perspective. I have tried to organize the discussions on the topics which do not find frequent mention in other books. I believe that we can't understand despair, guilt, or anxiety until we acknowledge the interdependent domains of their origins. Building a sustainable world is no easy task only of the psychologists, and we need our personal honesty, academic vision, courage, and commitment to do it. I have tried to point out real-life experiences and wrote this book to be an alternative tool as well as textbook for mental health and well-being. This book has taught me a great deal while developing some degrees of consciousness about the complexity of its vastness.

Acknowledgements

There are so many people to thank who generally contributed their help to shape nuances of this journey. In this regard, I especially express my unfathomable thanks to my wife Swati, who helped me realize that I am capable for doing it. I am deeply indebted to my teachers, colleagues, friends, and family who have helped me to achieve this herculean task. I am very grateful to Prof. Girishwar Mishra, Prof. Anand Prakash, Prof. R.B. Solanki, Prof. Ritesh Singh, Prof. Purnima Singh, Dr. Abraham P.F., Prof. Seema Aleem, Prof. Ghazi Shahnawaz, Prof. P.K. Mishra, Prof. Naved Iqbal, Prof. N.K. Chadha, Prof. Sanjay Srivastava, Prof. Roopali Sharma, and Prof. Sarita Roy for their contribution to my thinking and motivation.

I am also very grateful for the support and friendship of my colleagues across Delhi University, Department of Psychology, and other universities.

I also wish to thank all my college undergraduate students.

There is no doubt that the long period of time during which this book has been in preparation, which must have seemed especially protracted to my family, went away smoothly for their love, forbearance support, and sacrifices. In this regard, I express my unfathomable thanks to my wife for her boundless encouragement and patience, helping me realize that I am capable of doing it. I also thank my son Kanishk for tolerating my period of solitude and preoccupation with his evergreen smile and my daughter Kriti who did something meaningful and kept me energized throughout the preparation of the manuscript.

The book began and was completed with investments of many people. I am indebted to friends and colleagues who encouraged me to write this book. I wish to thank the teachers who always encouraged me with steadfast support. More things in the world are accomplished by groups rather than by single individuals working alone. I am blessed to have been part of many wonderful groups in my life time. I should also like to express my gratitude to my family friends J.K. Mishra, Ashok Kumar, Vivek Deep, Dharmendra, and Somendra. I also wish to express my gratitude to Sh. Surendra Kumar ji, Uday Sahay ji, Tajender Luthra ji, Suman Nalwa ji undergraduate student, Praveer Ranjan ji, Ajay Narain ji, Deepak Kumar, Rishiraj ji, Prabodh Chandra ji, Kumar Hrishikesh ji, Amaresh Singh ji,

Faisal Sulaiman, Sanjay Mandal, Prashant Kumar, Malay Neerav, Rajnish Kumar, Sanjeev Roy, Dr Jaikishore, Dr Ravi Malik, Atulya Sharma, Bidhan Chandra, Deepa, and Samyak.

I offer my sincere praise to my family members, especially my elder brother Sh. L.P. Singh, Manoj, Savita, Rudra, Asmita, Pushkar, Anushka, Piyush, Kunal, Aman, Tripurari, Ashok, Prashant, and Sanjay K. Singh for their unconditional love and emotional support throughout the journey. Finally, I dedicate this work to my Mother and my Father Late Sh. C.B. Singh.

1 Mental Health and Well-being

Learning Objectives

After reading this chapter, you will be able to understand

- Mental health and well-being
- Stress and coping
- Influencers of well-being (ecology, work–life, Indian and Western perspectives, culture and spirituality)

Introduction

Mental health and well-being constitute one of the most relevant areas in the discipline of psychology, and, despite significant researches, these concepts are so broad and interdisciplinary in scope that they cannot be confined to the narrow boundary of psychology alone.

Mental health is no longer a static set of characteristics limited to the domain of psychology. Rather, a set of factors contributing to the mind–body–soul harmony and a holistic paradigm of thinking are required for a comprehensive understanding of this subject.

The notion of mental health and well-being has evolved historically with the change of traditions, cultures, and technological developments.

The concept of mental health can be typically explained with the help of physiological, emotional, psychological, and social determinants. It is very rare that clinical psychologists and psychiatrists tend to explore factors like air quality, water quality, the locale of one's residences, neighbourhood, fauna and flora, drainage system, cultural systems, spiritual practices, and overall civilizational human virtues in their diagnosis of mental health issues.

Mental health and wellness are determined by a complex interplay of demographic factors, cultural influences, physical environment, social influences, the policies of the government, industrialization of the society, spiritual orientation, civic virtues, work–life balance, excessive use of the Internet, family environment, values in the society, economic loss, human

DOI: 10.4324/9781003350651-1

rights, and many other less discussed and highlighted arenas. It is crucial to point out the relational process of establishing a harmony with a broader context of human reality and nature's reality.

The traditional approach of clinical psychology perspective of treating mental health problems from a binary perspective of illness and treatment is not a realistic way of approaching this issue.

Historical Antecedents

The whole of human civilization has been intrigued by the term 'insanity', and various belief systems influenced cultural and behavioural practices. It was believed in earlier times that insanity might cause wolf-madness, a disease which a person is said to be suffering from when they prowl about graves and pray at the moon (Porter, 2002). It is strange to highlight that as long as till fourteenth century, people suspected of being werewolves were hunted and executed throughout Europe. Perhaps, lycanthropy or wolf-madness was one of the earliest diagnoses of melancholy.

Mental illness was extensively studied by Persian scholars during the period between ninth and twelfth centuries AD, which was also known as the Golden Age of Islamic Medicine. Muhammad ibn Zakariya al-Razi (865–925 AD) was an influential Persian physician considered among the first in the world to write on mental illness and psychotherapy.

Trephining is considered to be one of the earliest surgical methods to alleviate the suffering of individuals with mental disorders. Medical instruments in Greece and Rome confirmed that surgeons continued the practices of perforating cranium between 25 BC and 216 AD (Faria, 2013). In the ancient times, people having committed crimes were treated like outcasts, and they were killed in many situations. Hippocrates (c. 460–357 BC), the father of medicine, believed that mental illness was an organic sickness not caused by demons. It was suggested according to Hippocratic belief that medicine should be practiced as a scientific inquiry to understand the disease symptoms with the knowledge of anatomy.

Soranus of Ephesus, a Greek physician living in Rome during the second century AD, argued about the Methodist (or medical thinking) school of physicians (Kleisiaris et al., 2014). The believers of this school treated approached individuals with care and compassion. As per the new testament of Christian Bible, expulsion of demonic spirits through Exorcism occurs when a demon is commanded by a priest in the name of God to stop his activity within a person (Baglio, 2010). Exorcism to expel evil is still a part of religious beliefs around the world.

In 500 BC, Siddhartha Gautama, later known as Gautam Buddha in the world, pioneered Buddhism on the basis of the principle that the origin of mental suffering is ignorance, and its major causes are attachment and craving which can be cured by following the eightfold path of Buddhism.

In the tenth century AD, Ahmed ibn Sahl al-Balkhi (Balkh Afghanistan) introduced the concepts of mental health also recognizing the fact that illnesses can have both psychological and/or physiological causes.

Abu-Alial-Hussyn-Ibn Abdalah ibn-Sina (980–1030 AD), known to the west as Avicenna, in his legendary work, the Canon of medicine (Al-Qanun-fit-il-Tabb), provided rich description and treatments for insomnia, mania, vertigo, paralysis, epilepsy, depression, and mate sexual dysfunctions (Mahdi et al., 1987).

One of the most influential Sufi psychologists was Al-Ghazali (1058–111 AD), a prolific author and regarded as one of the greatest thinkers of Islam. He argued about the concepts of knowledge of self-knowledge of God, knowledge of the world, and knowledge of the future world. He wrote a celebrated masterpiece: *Kiniya-yi-Saada* (*Alchemy of Happiness,* approximately around 1105 AD). *Alchemy of Happiness* prescribed methods of self-discipline and asceticism. Due to its spiritual dimensions, *Kiniya* is considered to be the noblest of all occult sciences. *Nafs* is an Arabic word occurring in *Quran,* literally meaning self also translated as psyches ego or soul. There are three principal stages of *nafs* in a Sufi wisdom in the processes of development, retirement, and mastery of the *nafs*.

Johann Weyer (1515–88) is recognized as the first physician to specialize in the treatment of mental illness 'melancholy', as it was then termed (Cavanaugh, 2015). Weyer is considered as the founder of modern psychiatry, and he was opposed to the practice of punishing or killing suspected witches. He further argued that most confessions to practising witchcraft were made under the duress of coercion, and hence were unreliable. Witches were suspected to have supernatural powers, and witch hunt claimed millions of lives over the next 250 years officially began during 1400s (Cavanaugh, 2015).

Other notable and landmarks in the field of mental health diagnosis and treatment include the work of Phillipe Pinel who published *Treatise on Insanity* (1806), and Jean-martin Charcot (1984) explained demonic possession as a form of hysteria (conversion disorder) to be treated with hypnotherapy. Sigmund Freud's work interpretation of dreams (1900) marked the beginning of psychoanalytic thought. Carl Jung initially associated with Freud's work but later founded a new school of thought known as analytical psychology.

Michael Foucault categorized society's responses to mental illness into three distinct periods of time (Foucault, 2009). The first age of Renaissance represented a time period when madness was considered to be the reverse of wisdom, in the years between fourteenth and seventeenth centuries. This stage is followed by Classical Age in seventeenth to eighteenth centuries, a time when confinement was used as a way to control mental illness. The third stage is known as Modern Age, which was towards the end of eighteenth century, which considered mental illness as an object of scientific scrutiny as a disease to be controlled. The term phrenology originally derived from Greek word *mind* means that brain is composed of separate organs, each of which corresponds to a skill controlled by the human mind. In his 1916 edition of *Mental Disorders of Men,* Bernard Hollander argued that nervous conditions were a socially induced phenomena, attributing the increase in mental illness to be a consequence of progress in civilization. In his 1916 book, *Nervous Disorders of Men*, Hollander concluded that women were more prone to nervous disorders than men. He further stated that one reason for the mental disorders women experience was that 'they typically had foolish desires to be regarded as somebody of value in society' (Hollander, 2015).

The foundation of American Psychological Association headed by G. Stanley Hall in 1892, was a crucial juncture in the field of psychology. In 1913, Jacob L. Moreno applied group psychotherapy methods in Vienna.

The context of industrialization and rising labour problems with the additional rise in urbanity phenomenon led to the acceptance of mental problems, which were noted as organic physical phenomena. During the earlier times, people with mental issues were considered strange and stigmatized elements of the society, and treatment of such people involved barbaric practices.

The end of nineteenth century AD and the beginning of twentieth century witnessed several developments that could strengthen the initiatives taken towards improving mental health and wellness.

Carl Jung and Carl Roger's journal contribution related to client-centred therapy, Gestalt therapy work pioneered by Fritz et al., rational emotive therapy by Albert Ellis, and Victor Frankl's work on men's search for meaning were other significant contributions in the field of mental illness and mental health.

One of the most systematic and landmark development was the establishment of Diagnostic Statistical Manual of Mental Disorders published by American Psychiatric Association, marking the beginning of modern mental illness classification.

The theory by Thomas Szasz was directed toward anti-psychiatry movement, and his concept of myths of mental illness allowed the exploration of diverse dimensions of mental health and wellness.

Several other thoughts, theories, and researches in the field of mental illness and mental health included Hermann Rorschach's inkblot test, Sir Henry Dale's discovery of acetylcholine, and Julius Jauregg's invention of malarial therapy for the treatment of general paralysis of the insane.

The era of psychopharmacology promoted the use of anti-psychotic drugs for the treatment of mentally ill people. Some of the medicines prescribed by psychiatrics acquired a universal recognition for the treatment of mental health problems.

India's Contribution to the Field of Mental Health

India's contribution to the field of mental health had been remarkable. *Charak Samhita* is a Sanskrit text on Indian traditional medicine. Though there is ambiguity on the exact date, its tentative compilation is considered to be held around fourth to second century BC by a number of scholars, prominent among which are Atreya, Agnivesha Charaka, and Dridhbala.

Charak is a Sanskrit term for a wanderer or Sanyasi (ascetic), and it is used to denote the knowledge of wandering physicians.

Atharva Veda texts argued that life is of four kinds, which are *Sukha* (Happy), *Dukha* (unhappy), *Hita* (good), and *Ahita* (bad).

Charak Samhita uses the fundamental assumptions of *Vedas* which mention that humans are micro replicas of the universe which comprises theory of six elements (five *Prakriti* and one *Brahmin*), three humours (*Vata*, *Pitta*, and *Kapha*), and three *guna* (*Sattva*, *Rajas*, and *Tamas*) as constituting factors innately present in a human body.

During the reign of king Ashoka, many hospitals for patients with mental illness were built according to the scribes of *Ashoka Samhita*.

The earliest mental hospital in India was established at Bombay in 1745, which was made to accommodate approximately 30 mentally ill patients.

The first government-run lunatic asylum was opened on 17th April 1795 at Monghyr (later known as Munger) in Bihar, especially for insane soldiers. Under the Indian Lunacy Act 1912, a European lunatic asylum was established in Bhawanipore for European patients which was closed down after the establishment of the European Hospital at Ranchi in 1918. The origins of psychiatric rehabilitation in India can be traced back with the establishment of CIP (Central Institute of Psychiatry in 1922) which got its affiliation from the University of London to start diploma in psychological medicine.

The first drafts of Mental Health Act of India (1987) was written at Ranchi in 1949. Research in psychiatry began with the publication of first journal dedicated to mental health: the 'Indian Journal of Neurology and Psychiatry in 1949'. A formal training program for clinical psychologists (Diploma in Medical Psychology) commenced at NIMHANS in the year 1955 and was later converted into an M.Phil. degree in Medical and Social Psychology in 1978. Girindra Shekhar Bose founded the Indian Psychoanalytical Association in 1922 in Calcutta (Nizamie & Goyal, 2010).

Current Scenario of Mental Health Problem in the World and India

World Mental Health Day is observed on 10th October every year with the objective of raising awareness about mental health issues and for the enhancement of effective strategies for promoting mental health. Mental and behavioural disorders are the result of a complex interaction between biological, psychological, social, and cultural factors.

The clinical description and diagnostic guidelines for ICD-10 mental and behavioural disorder are listed as 'a clinically recognizable set of symptoms or behaviours associated in most cases with distress and with interference with personal functions'.

The International Classification of Disorders (ICD) is an international standard diagnostic classification for a wide variety of health conditions produced by World Health Organization (WHO). The chapter V of ICD-10 focuses on mental and behavioural disorders which consists of ten groups, and these are:

- F_1 – Organic, including symptomatic, mental disorders:
- F_2 – Mental and behavioural disorders due to the use of psychoactive substances
- F_3 – Schizophrenia
- F_4 – Mood [affective] disorders
- F_5 – Neurotic disorders
- F_6 – Behavioural syndromes associated with physiological and physical disturbances
- F_7 – Disorders of personality and behaviour in adult people
- F_8 – Mental retardation
- F_9 – Disorders of psychological development
- F_{10} – Behavioural and emotional disorders in childhood and adolescences.

In addition, a group of unspecified mental disorders is also included in this classification.

The classification of mental disorders is also known as psychiatric nosology, and two most established systems for classifying mental disorders are ICD-10 produced by WHO and DSM produced by American Psychological Association.

ICD is a categorical classification system whereas DSM is a dimensional approach to classification.

The Diagnostic and Statistical Manual Mental Disorder (DSM, later edition was DSM-5 published in 2013) has significant changes in the fifth edition through the detection of sub-types of schizophrenia-paranoid, disorganized catatonic, undifferentiated, and residual. The detection of the subsets of autistic spectrum disorder – namely, Asperger's syndrome, Classic autism, Rett syndrome, childhood disintegrative disorder, and pervasive developmental disorder not otherwise specified – was also implemented with indications of intensity that were mild, moderate, and severe.

In recent years, there has been an increasing acknowledgement of the mental health problems, and WHO started special initiatives for the improvement of mental health and depression was one of the priority areas to be covered by WHO's Mental Health Gap Action Programme (MhGAP, 2008). Other mental disorders WHO report of 2001 regarding the prevalence of disorders suggested 450 million people estimated to be suffering from neuropsychiatric conditions.

Surveys conducted in developed as well as developing countries have shown that during their entire lifetime, more than 25% of individuals develop one or more mental or behavioural disorders (Regier et al., 1988; Wells et al., 1889; Almeida-Filho et al., 1997).

Mental disorders are among the leading causes of non-fatal disease burden in India. In the Global Burden of Disease study (1990–2017), prevalence of mental disorders, years lived with disability (YEDS), and disability-adjusted life-years (DALYS) caused by twelve factors in India from 1990 to 2017 was evaluated. In this study, 127.3 million people had mental disorders in India, including 45.7 million with depressive disorders and 44.5 million with anxiety disorders in the year 2017.

In 2017, depressive disorders contributed the most to the total number of mental disorders: DALYS (33.8%), followed by anxiety disorders (19%), idiopathic developmental intellectual disability (IDID 10.8%), schizophrenia (8.8%), bipolar disorder (6.9%), conduct disorders (5.9%), autism spectrum disorders (3.2%), eating disorders (2.2%), attention deficit hyperactivity disorder (0.3%), and other mental disorders comprised 8% of DALYS.

The intensity of prevalence was higher in states with low socio-demographic index (SDI) than in middle SDI and high SDI states in 2017.

It was estimated through this report that one in seven Indians were affected by mental disorders of varying severity in 2017. There have been substantial variations across states, but the proportional contribution of mental disorders to the total disease burden in India has almost doubled since 1990. India launched its first mental health policy in 2014 and revised Mental Health Care Act in 2017 with the objective of providing effective and universal access to mental healthcare.

National Mental Health Survey of India (2015–16) conducted by NIMHANS Bangalore and supported by the Ministry of Health and Family Welfare estimated the prevalence and pattern of various mental disorders in a representative Indian population.

The NIMHANS report suggests that nearly fifteen percent of Indian adults are in need of active intervention with one or the other mental disorder.

According to the findings of this report, prominent mental health problems in an Indian context include autism among children, depression among pregnant women and youth, and the problem of dementia among the elderly population. Bipolar affective disorder is more prevalent among urban males owing to lifestyle and other problems.

A nation's culture, values mental healthcare services significantly impacts its population's mental health sometimes the prevalence is most actually manifested owing to the stigma attached with screening for mental health.

Finland tops in UN's happiness rankings, but it is not free from all aspects and its substance abuse and adolescent depression and suicide rates are well beyond the European average.

Afghanistan has an abnormally high rate of depression owing to decades of armed conflict and economic misery, but some of the affluent countries' people are also depressed, making it a complex phenomenon. It is also suggested that it is a culture of pessimism which is responsible for depression not the poverty alone, and it is sometimes said that people in poor countries do not have the leisure to be depressed.

Mental Illness to Mental Health

The influences of labelling, stigma, categorization, and prejudice are some of the important attitudes distancing mentally ill patients from seeking help and treatment.

Many expletives used in our day-to-day life activities such as 'are you insane' and 'have you gone mad' convey stereotype and stigma regarding mental illness. The organized category of stigma and broader social rejection accentuate a sense of role failure in mentally ill patients.

The mentally ill patients suffering from problems have feelings of shame and silencing, which further create a paradoxical situation of having dual disadvantages at individual and social levels.

Think Box

1. What is your opinion about the mental health profession?
2. What are the impediments in the growth of mental health infrastructure in India?

Mental health and mental illness are related phenomena of a continuing spectrum as the effects of ongoing stress on mental health can lead to mental illness if left unchallenged. Stigma is a universal phenomenon which poses severe restrictions and discriminations for the mentally ill patients. Stigma can be described on the bases of physical, social, and mental types.

However, recent developments were related to sensitivity and awareness of mental health problems with sustained efforts by mental health professionals. Social workers and government initiatives have resulted in fostering a positive attitude towards them.

Parental initiatives, community support, and digital media platforms have contributed to demystify the myth around mental illness, which have led to the frank disclosure of mental health problems and their gradual acceptance by the society.

The pioneers of positive psychology approach have focused upon the factors of hope, optimism, self-efficacy, and resilience which resulted in the growth of positive emotions and well-being. The growth perspective of mental health depends on the realization of human potential through lifestyle changes.

The traits of optimism and hope relate positively with better mental health state. The role of supportive relationships and that of positive interaction between family, friends, and significant others contribute to the well-being of the people.

Stress and Coping

Prior to industrialization, the nature of societies was largely governed by man-made mediations of relationships on the basis of face-to-face interactions with sharing of strong social bonds.

The rapid advancements in technology, urbanization, lifestyle problems, and rise of consumerism have led to a rise in the levels of stress at individual and community levels. The chapter on stress and coping will explore the impact of modernity, technology, and capitalism on the lives of people and its resultant consequences of stress.

In order to achieve the individualistic goals and high-edge competitiveness, people conflicts at intrapersonal, interpersonal, and professional levels have increased, and stress has acquired the form of an epidemic in modern times. The causes of stress in eastern and Western perspectives have slightly different orientations. In the eastern perspective, stress results from a lack of balance between inner and outer world realities, whereas in the Western perspective, outer material pursuits are accorded greater importance.

The important factors discussed in the theories of psychology include physiological, personality, social, and professional dimensions of stress. People experiencing stress about their existing state of affairs may experience physical and psychological symptoms such as irritability, anger, fatigue, and difficulty in sleeping. Stress has become a very common determinant in modern-day life activities which may arise due to work, family, financial difficulties, unemployment, and other social circumstances. It is also important to realize that individuals vary a lot in adapting to demanding situations guided by factors of age, economic status, and support mechanisms available to them.

The origin of stress may be psychogenic, biogenic, or contextual, adversely affecting the individual's well-being.

The cognitive approach focuses on the subjective interpretation made by an individual in response to a stimulus in the environment. The environment and the transactional or interactional orientation focus more on thoughts that impact the overall individual stress response an individual can have in his or her mind and body. The transactional approach focuses more upon cognitions and perceptions which mediate the response to stressful events. From the cognitive perspective, an individual's interpretation of the environment plays a crucial role in the elicitation of the stress response. The chapter on stress and coping will help to understand various conceptualizations of stress and coping and their relationships with health and well-being. Life events of an individual demand adjustment across various dimensions, and positive approaches in life can lead towards wellness. The importance of the socio-cultural context and its role are very crucial is turning stressful situations into wellness. Indian approach of handling stressful situations offers diverse advantages in terms of its collectivistic orientation towards life and joint family system that provide better support system to improve well-being. Community traditions of participation in social activities and rituals can foster a positive climate for navigating life in a meaningful way. Health-care proponents suggest a fundamentally changed perspective from diagnosis and treatment of illness to the measurement and delivery of wellness.

The ecological context, social context, spiritual context, and understanding the nature of suffering and healing are important contributors to the problems of mental health in an increasingly complex and globalized society. The chapter on stress and coping provides rich theoretical and empirical description and analyses their implications on mental health.

Ecology and Well-being

The chapter on ecology and well-being deals with the importance of the issues of ecological contexts in supporting social and emotional development of people. The chapter explores ecological context analysis of well-being as an investigation of the relationships among individuals, others, and their physical surroundings. Ecological perspective is a process of understanding how individual's experiences contribute to 'making sense' of situations and experiences negotiated progressively over time and place. An ecological analysis of well-being provides an opportunity to investigate multi-directional-interactions and its influence on the well-being of an individual.

The theoretical and empirical evidences have been summarized to highlight the importance of observing an individual within the context of the multiple environments in which they are positioned.

The ecosystem approach is a strategy for integrating and managing natural resources and human resources which can promote conservation and sustainable use in an equitable manner. The objective of ecosystem approach is to protect the inhabitants of the earth from potential harm or damage to planet. Ecosystem approach involves a wide range of activities to increase the resilience and reduce threats to people due to environmental and climatic changes. The process of ecosystem management interest of some stakeholders should not pose harmful effects to other ecosystems.

Planet earth is undergoing rapid environmental changes because of human actions. Humans have destroyed a large portion of some types of ecosystems. Pollutions of air and water are a major source of ill-health including their adverse effects on reproductive health. The culture of consumption leads to higher levels of production, which generate larger quantities of waste. The term 'anthropogenic' designates an effect or object resulting from human activity. The term 'anthropocene' is used in the context of pollution emissions that have been produced from the activities since the beginning of agricultural revolution, and it broadly applies to all major human impacts on the environment. According to the first law of thermodynamics, the total energy of an isolated system is constant, energy can be transformed from one form to another, but can be neither created nor destroyed.

According to second law of thermodynamics, an order can be increased within a system (such as human economy) only by increasing disorder or entropy outside the system (i.e. the environment). Hence, technological advancements can create order in the economy at the expense of increasing disorder in the environment. Defaunation, the loss of animals from ecological communities, is being caused by profligate consumption and human overpopulation.

The concept of paradox of plankton results from the conflict between the observed diversity of plankton and the competitive exclusion principle stating that when two species compete for the same resource, finally, only one will survive. This paradox can be resolved by the factors of symbiosis, differential predation, and spatio-temporal heterogeneity.

The importance of wellness in fostering wellness and mental health has been found to be very effective. Evidence from positive psychologists and researches of emotions continue to suggest that life-well-being indications can be measured and improved. Positive emotions improve an individual's well-being and significantly affect the mental-health conditions of the people.

The term 'quality of life' is similar to psycho-social well-being which involves emotional, social, and psychological dimensions.

This chapter on ecological well-being and mental health will present the concepts and researches on relationships between ecological varieties and mental health. The concept of psycho-social well-being has received considerable interest in recent years within the scientific and psychology literature. Increasing evidence suggest that psychological well-being (PWB) is associated with lower disease and mortality risk which can be improved with the help of interventions. Distinct theoretical dimensions characterizing psychological well-being include hedonic well-being (e.g. feeling happy), evaluative well-being (e.g. being satisfied with life), and eudaimonic well-being (e.g. finding purpose in life, having a sense of mastery and autonomy in one's own decisions), and other constructs of hope and opinions can contribute to feeling of wellness.

Indian context of wellness and ecological well-being suggests that people's desires include *dharma* (virtue), *artha* (wealth), *kama* (pleasure), and *moksha* (liberation), which are called *purushartha* (human values); and a Sanskrit term for happiness or wellness is *ananda,* which is the nearest to English 'bliss' that is associated with spirituality.

According to the ancient Indian perspective, *dharma* is based on four major factors that is i) *desa* (place, region), (ii) *kal* (time), (iii) karma (action), and (iv) *guna* (natural traits).

Think Box

Critically discuss the role of interdisciplinary approach for mental health and well-being.

The concept of *deoban* (sacred forests) attaches deity status to forest, and it is preserved through community participation. Indian mythological texts consider space, air, fire, water, and earth as the foundations of an interconnected web of life. *Upanishads* explain the interdependence of five elements of existence in relation to Brahman, the supreme reality from which they arise 'From Brahman arises space, from space arises air, from air arises fire, from fire arises water and from water arises earth'. People in Indian tradition revere rivers such as the Ganges as goddess, also described as Ma Ganga or 'Mother Ganges'. A number of rural Hindu communities such as Bishnois, Bhils, and Swadhyaya have maintained strong emotional connect and spiritualties within the forests and animals till date. The Chipko movement made famous by Chipko women's commitment to 'hugging' trees in their community to protect them from felling by outside interests represents a devotion to the forests as being sacred. It is a very common practice in India offering devotional rituals to trees of Amla, Peepal, Tulsi, and many others and praying and giving god-like respects to them. An important Hindu festival, Chatt Puja, is celebrated in which millions of devotees recite prayers to the evening sun, offering prayers to the rising sun with the chanting of mantras. The worship is performed for the welfare of the world. Such type of integral traditional ceremonies, rituals, and sacrifices clearly indicate strong human nature handing in the Indian context. Special texts based on *Ahimsa* (non-violence), the practice of not causing injury to other living creatures, are integral to Indian tradition. The chapter on health and well-being will cover the details of theories and researches related to coping.

Work–Life Well-being

The problem of workplace stress has led to new fields of psychological study – occupational health psychology concerned with occupation and employee well-being. The goal of occupational health psychology is to understand and combat the harmful effects of stress on employee health and safety.

The effects of job pressure are not same for all the employees, and all the stresses are not considered to be harmful. The work–life balance results in high job satisfaction leading to good health and longevity. In most of the explanations related to personality aspects, type A personality people are highly competitively driven, with a constant sense of time urgency, which is often associated with problems like heart disease, anger hostility, time urgency, and depression. Type B personality persons may be ambitious but experience less stress at work and have fewer stress effects. Another personality variable that can play a crucial role resulting in individual differences in showing vulnerability to stress is hardiness. Hardiness factor allows persons to have more self-belief and self-control over the events in their lives, hence they are more resistant to stress. Personality factors such as self-efficacy, locus of control, and self-esteem may also contribute to the variations in the experience of stress in working conditions.

A poor work–life balance can lead to a variety of symptoms which can effect an employee's well-being. The time between work and life has been the subject of interest among scholars and researchers. The concept of work–life balance has acquired importance as it plays a crucial role in improving the productivity of organizations and their people. Positive work–life conditions lead to increased satisfaction whereas negative or stressful work–life balance can lead to failure in performing tasks, getting turnovers, and showing absenteeism. The notion of harmony and equilibrium between family life and professional life is emphasized to achieve overall productivity.

Work–life balance is not a static process, and effective interventions can improve the balance of role-related expectations in professional and family arena.

A large variety of factors such as engagements, flow, and organizational commitment contribute positively to maintain the balance. Similarly, employee performance and affective organizational commitment help individuals to have more satisfaction in their work.

Positive psychology argues about the context of positive organizational scholarship focused upon the study of positive outcomes, processes, and attributes of organizations and their members.

Work–life balance equilibrium is supported by the concepts of happiness and achievement. The balancing process of self, family, society, and organization can be improved by reducing conflicts in these domains. Setting one's priorities, finding a job that one likes to do, attention to health, spending time with loved ones, and setting boundaries for oneself are some of the important steps suggested to achieve the work–life balance.

However, in reality, there are no clear prescriptions so that one can easily practice achieving work–life well-being. Demographic factors, attitudinal factors, and situational factors also play an important role in it. Indian perspective of work is a form of worship, where no work is superior or inferior in nature. Lord Krishna advises his disciple Arjuna to perform every action with a spirit of devotion for common welfare. Work done with a spiritual attitude leads to an expansion of mind and soul. Sri Krishna said 'karmanyaevadhikaraste ma phaleshukadachanama-karma-phala-heturbhur ma tesango 'Stvakarmani" (the *Bhagavad Gita*, Chapter Two, verse 47). This roughly means that 'You have the right to perform your prescribed duty, but you are not entitled to the fruits of action. Never consider yourself the cause of the results of your activities and never be attached to not doing your duty.

When the work is done with the spirit of worship of God, it is called Karmayoga, done with devotion and purity. The fruit of your work belongs solely to the Lord of all works. The attachment to the fruit of work, considered to be the faults of ego, and the sense of doer ship have to be relinquished. The chapter on work–life balance and well-being brings a number of fundamental concepts, questions, and empirical researches to identify its direct and indirect implications on mental health and well-being.

Culture and Well-being

The chapter on culture and well-being provides a rich idea about culturally patterned interests, motivations, and behavioural implications. The conception of interdependence of society, culture, and mental health has many implications for each other. I hope it will become evident to the readers that this inquiry into the interdependence of different spheres plays a crucial role in the development of mental health and well-being.

In the last few years, there has been a growing understanding of the impact that culture and cultural diversity can have on health and well-being. There are a variety of definitions of culture from sociological, psychological, and anthropological points of view. Culture consists of ideas and things that are passed on from one generation to the next in a society which includes knowledge, beliefs, values, customs, symbols, and material products that help member of a society to meet human needs. There are important social and legitimate institutions, religious institutions, and economic and political institutions which help its members to share a common culture. Norms concerning behaviours of the members may be strict or moderate carrying powerful sanctions. A woman who becomes pregnant outside marriage is condemned in certain societies, and her children bear the stigma of being illegitimate. Norms of a culture are classified into three categories of folkways, mores, and laws based largely on how important are the norms in the society and people's response to the breach of such norms. The conflicts between different aspects of culture such as material culture, non-material culture, ideal culture, and real culture and values associated with them pose opportunities and threats to its members which can influence their well-being. The tendency to view one's own group and its cultural expectation to be right and proper and superior to others is called enthocentricism. People violating the culture taboo may be stigmatized and punished by other members of the same culture. Cultural relativism suggests setting aside personal beliefs and prejudice and appreciate the members of other cultural groups from their perspective only.

Durkheim described the concepts of mechanical solidarity in which members of pre-modern society were tied to common beliefs, values, emotional ties, and organic solidarity in which social positions are specialized and interdependent.

United Nations in its conference on cultural diversity highlighted the importance of affirming the respect for the tolerance of diversity of cultures, dialogue, and co-operation among members of different cultures.

Cultural pluralism helps to ensure harmonious interaction among people and groups with plural, varied, and dynamic cultural identities [UNESCO General Conference 2nd Nov. 2001].

Subjective well-being is a complex and multifaceted concept, and it includes the combination of feeling good and functioning well.

A large body of literature also discusses the positive impacts of cultural activities on well-being. The chapter on culture and well-being will focus on facts which are barriers to cultural advantages and disadvantages that can improve or decrease well-being.

The Indian culture and traditions have the unique characteristics of reflecting collectivistic orientation; well-being of others (*paropkar*); good actions and bad actions (*dharmik* and *adharmik*); and balance in life between *dharma*, *artha*, and *kama* (duties, wealth, and pleasure).

A strong tendency of fasting rituals, respect to the elders, and focus on minimization of needs are characteristics of Indian culture. The concept of true happiness lies in maintaining a harmony of spirit, mind, and body. The concept of *Vasudhaiva Kutumbakam* (the world as one family) clearly highlights the broader connectivity orientation of Indian culture.

Spirituality and Well-being

Spirituality is used to denote the experiential and personal side of our relationships with the transcendent or sacred.

Spirituality comprises central themes which include values and ultimate meaning beyond self, a way of understanding, awareness, and personal integration. It also contains some elements of mysteriousness.

The chapter of spirituality and well-being intends to view the role of spirituality in the domain of mental health. I shall examine the texture of theories that emerged in the field of spirituality and their critical role in the field of mental health and well-being. The model of spirituality provides an effective alternative with its enlarging and deepening impact on mental health and well-being. Today, the entire world appreciates the power of spirituality to resolve myriads of mental health problems. The emphasis on intrinsic rationale for transformation serves as a strategic and realistic addition to the field of mental health and well-being. The failure of modern science to foresee some of the most fundamental problems of our society can find a positive recovery in the realm of spirituality sphere.

Spirituality is considered to be a protective factor against a host of negative health outcomes. Characteristics of spirituality include meaning and value transcendence, connected with self and other's growth. Spirituality is also related to an individual's feelings about supreme power, hope, reduced sadness, and orientation towards helping others without expectations.

Spiritual health can affect physical, mental, and social aspects of health. Spiritual people have a disciplined lifestyle, which enhances health and well-being. Spiritual practices also promote mindfulness which is a key contributor to mental health initiatives. Spirituality involves considering perspectives and multiple truths in life. In mental health issues, the clients often experience identity- and meaning-related issues in which spirituality helps to discover one's identity through awareness and mindfulness practices.

The questions of existential nature such as 'Who am I?', 'Why I am here?', and 'Where do I fit in?' are related to identity, purpose, and place and are a part of the making meaning. Happiness and emotional well-being can be achieved through spiritual activities of awareness of self and others. Researchers have found that if spirituality is related with lifestyle, it can influence cognitive and affective activities.

The importance of spirituality is to provide a set of values and meanings, and meanings give order to the world. It is also evidenced through researches and studies that ideas about one's life and the world can help people to overcome stressful situations.

Spiritual identity of a person promotes the characteristics of spirituality in personal sense of self linked with well-being. A system of belief in certain transcendental goals provides a resource to overcome stressors. Frankl believed that a belief system may make life meaningful by giving man goals such as a purpose to achieve, rules to follow, and rituals and values which act as a protective layer against harming oneself.

When it comes to strategies related to reinterpreting difficult circumstances into meaningful ones, religiosity and spirituality have been seen to work as the main sources (Baumister).

Self-reflection, self-regulation, and self-growth are being positively correlated in the journey of a spiritual seeker, which have a positive impact on their well-being. Spiritual people tend to practise the altruistic and pro-social behavioural pattern which provides direct and indirect support to overcoming difficulties.

In the Indian perspective of spirituality, the harmony of spirit, mind, and body is emphasized. Indian spirituality is described through principles of *Vedas*, *Upanishads*, the *Bhagavad Gita,* and other mythological works. Buddhism and the philosophy of the *Bhagavad Gita* and Upanishads are not remote from popular Indians beliefs and everyday activities. In the Indian society, religion is not a dogma but a way of life, and human conduct with intimate relation between the truth of philosophy and the daily life of people makes religion more alive and less mystical. The spiritual dimensions of the Indian culture encompass in detail the topics of the nature of God, the end of life, and the relation of the individual to the universal soul. Indian spirituality makes philosophical attempts to know the inner truth, and 'Atmanam vidhi' that is a way to know the self sums up the laws of nature. From a psychological perspective, value of concentration is emphasized as a means for the perception of the truth, and concepts like telepathy and clairvoyance are neither considered abnormal nor miraculous. In the philosophy of Buddhism and its concept of Nirvana, six components of charity, virtue, patience, fortitude, meditation, and knowledge are especially mentioned. Buddhism prescribes practising a perfection of benevolence towards all living beings.

Suffering and Healing

The concept of stress denotes a feeling of pain which can affect the immunity and well-being of individuals.

Any event, experience, or environmental stimulus can cause stress in an individual, which can make them to be the causes of both physical and psychological problems. Different types of stressors can be classified into four categories – (a) catastrophes; (b) major life events (job, marriage, death of near ones, divorce); (c) daily hassles (work, office, deadlines); and (d) ambient stressors.

Psychological theories also suggest various types of conflicts namely – approach-approach conflict (happening due to two equally attractive options), avoidance-avoidance conflicts (occurs when a person chooses between two equally unattractive options); and approach-avoidance conflict (when a person is split between attractive and unattractive options). The ambient source of stressors may include the physical factors of noise, pollution, traffic congestion, difficulties in community, crowding, and so on. Organizational stressors may include difficult and threatening job conditions of military and combat field, toxic leadership, political turmoil in the country, and poor working conditions. Theories of stress enumerate various stress-causing factors and individual's resistance to counter them and a stage of exhaustion being reached, failing in the strategies for coping with them.

There are various strategies for coping suggested by researches, and important among them include use of humour, denial, rationalization, time management, attribution style changes, guided imagery time management, social support, and resilience building.

In the eastern perspective, suffering is considered as a life process made up of duality (happiness–pain or *sukh–dukh*) in almost all particulars of creation.

According to Buddhism, there are four unavoidable sufferings that are birth, old age, sickness, and death. There are three forms of mental sufferings: separation from people we love, contact with people we dislike, and frustration of desires. Suffering refers to psychological experience of profound that everything is impermanent, and the gap between reality and basic human tendency of life is *dukha* (suffering).

The ultimate causes of our suffering are greed, ignorance, and hatred which can lead to evil and anger. According to Jainism, causes of people's suffering are pointless generalizations, irrational scepticism, and ignorance known as *Mithyavada* (faulty assumptions). The tendency of *Aviroti* (non-restraint) is also a significant cause of our bondage. There are four important possessions of anger, pride, deceit, and greed which form the basis for the attachment of Karma to the soul. The concept of *Pramada* (carelessness and laxity of conduct) is caused due to absent mindedness and lack of spirit towards achieving spiritual growth.

According to the philosophy of the *Bhagavad Gita*, human suffering is real but not permanent. It is caused by faulty thinking, faulty perspectives, beliefs, and attitudes.

Majority of the people are suffering not because they are rich or poor, but because they have programmed their thoughts, desires, and actions to suffer. People also suffer due to false notions of identity, attachments, and lack of true knowledge. Hence, the understandings, perceptive, and thinking from broader perspective can offer us good mental health and well-being.

The chapter on suffering and well-being provides a detailed description of various mindfulness practices and their impact on well-being.

Critical Evaluation

A singular cause-and-effect perspective to understand, explore, and analyse the mental health and well-being will amount to a lopsided attempt in tackling this issue. A wider approach including micro, macro, and contextual dimensions needs to be analysed to gain better insights in understanding this subject.

Mental disorders are causal; they are always a result of some other causes. A strong tendency among professionals is to label people on the basis of misguided assumption. Majority of books on schizophrenia mention results of schizophrenia as being confused thinking, delusions, flat emotions, inappropriate behaviour, rambling, and so on; but in reality, schizophrenia rarely causes anything, rather they define schizophrenia on this basis.

For example influenza does not cause fever, headaches, and coughing, but the virus causes these symptoms. The symptoms in combination are labelled as influenza, and medication is provided to overcome the symptoms of fever, headache, and coughing, whereas in actuality, the medication that fights the virus itself and not just the symptoms should be given. A classic example of depression can help us understand the contradictory approach of medical model. Depression does not cause sadness, changes in sleep, appetite, low self-esteem, or suicidal thoughts. Life problems such as marriage of one's daughter, unemployment of children, poor economic condition, and social exclusion can be a cause of the symptoms labelled as depression.

A particular kind of ambiguous logic of faulty chemical imbalance is put forward by medical experts, which is lacking in terms of evidence. There are proofs that chemical imbalances affect human emotions, but human thinking, orientation towards life, and other life circumstances also alter chemistry of brain.

It is reasonable to suggest that brain chemistry must be considered in the context of social frameworks of motives, meanings, life stress, and spiritual orientation of a person. There are straightforward links of genetic diseases, and many environmental factors overlap profoundly with the disorders. Recent developments in the field of epigenetics are that genes themselves are affected and altered by the environment of their host.

Problems of each individual in the society dealing with daily life stressors, family, life condition, frustration in work–life balance, job identity crisis, overall conditions, and the resilience capacity of an individual to deal with crisis situations must be taken into account to determine the causes of mental disorders. It is also necessary to deconstruct the meanings of satisfaction one derives from work, ecology, culture, spiritual orientation, and his/her life orientation to adapt to and overcome those conditions. There is an urgent need to reconceptualize the entire dynamics of understanding of mental disorders as they are not static phenomena. It is fine to have a perspective as prescribed by Diagnostic Manual of Mental Illness, but to consider this as the only alternative will pose a formidable barrier to incorporate views and researches from cultural, social, spiritual, and personal origins.

People experiencing mental health problems also remain at the receiving end of stigma, inequality, injustice, and psycho-social alienation. There are several types of stigmas which are associated with mental distress and illness. These stigmas may include being the components of incompetence, danger to the society, and potential for committing violence. The concept of epistemic injustice which means harming someone by limiting his/her capacity to share knowledge is also a characteristic feature of people suffering from mental illness. Social isolation is a serious issue which people with mental illnesses have to face at individual, group, and larger social environment levels. It is argued that public has been duped in understanding the issues of mental health by making them believe that mental illnesses are scientifically validated bio-medical diseases. Mind is not a biological object like brain, rather it is riddled with elements of values, beliefs, assumption, desires, and doubts.

There are no fixed boundaries between normal variations and psychiatric boundaries, and a number of problems designated as mental illness are the results of professional endorsement, public consent, and doctrinal compliance to the labels. The splitting of psychological problems into mental illness category is a socio-cultural process not a scientific endeavour. Variety of issues like multiple personality disorder, homosexuality, general anxiety, and masturbation considered serious problems at some points in time are out of diagnostic manuals. The primary quality of brain is its complex physical structure, whereas the primary quality of mind is its complex intentionality, hence unsuitable for analysis on objective parameters. Majority of the scientific journals promote the idea for treating mental illness problems with doses of medication like other diseases. The so-called mental illness problems are treated at par with other biological diseases like pneumonia.

The point that seems to be less highlighted or unexplained in the Western model is undermining the impact of cultural context. Some of the crucial aspects of culture, societal norms, and spirituality can play a very significant role in deciding the mental health of an individual.

The dominant paradigms in the psychiatric diagnostic manuals are descriptions of mental states and behaviours regarded as symptoms, classification of those symptoms in graphs known as syndromes, and the diagnostic manuals to specify the causes of such syndromes, and an attempt is made to portray mental disorder in a naturalistic framework. For example the cause of depression among youth is suggested to be biological pathology, but factors like expectations, desires, values, role of social media, consumerism, and deficiency in education system are easily ignored, hence a lopsided analysis is presented. Life circumstances, cultural background, spiritual orientation, social environment, and political environment play an important role highlighting the dynamic nature of mental health problems. To claim that mental health problems like schizophrenia are caused only due to neurological and chemical imbalance is a simplistic reductionist error. The role of external factors like prolonged trouble in family setting and disturbingly ambiguous social environment and childhood environment can't be ruled out easily. This tendency to individualize the mental illness problems on the biological basis effectively cuts the link that had been discovered between disorders in children and bad parenting methods and other traumatic experiences during childhood.

Summary

This chapter on introduction to mental health and well-being is intended to incorporate several components. Primarily, this chapter brings together the notions of mental health and well-being. The section on historical antecedents focuses on the emergence of mental health issues from ancient period to contemporary times. It further highlights the response of the society to mental illness. This chapter also highlights the emergence of mental health issues and well-being in the Indian context. It attempts to provide a description of transition from good mental health to illness. Mental health and well-being are correlated to each other on a spectrum of continuity. The emphasis is placed on the interdependent determinants of mental health and well-being. The chapter introduces the readers to the implications of mental health from relevant constituents. The stress and coping are strongly related to the concept of mental health and well-being. This section focused on anticipated and unanticipated consequences of stress and coping on mental health. This chapter has only touched upon the fundamental contributions of stress and well-being, and rich descriptions have been provided in separate chapters. The critical overviews of ecology and well-being have been presented in this chapter. The character of this section is dictated by the twin circumstances that few theoretical questions have addressed to the phenomenon of ecology and well-being. The chapter has dealt with the concept of ecology and well-being in the Indian context as well.

In the subsequent section on work–life balance, questions like how much work is good work are discussed, along with the brief explanation of the rationale for work–life balance. Mainstream theories and texts strangely put less attention to such fundamental concepts of mental health and well-being.

Another section on culture and well-being deals with the complexities of the field without overwhelming or intimidating its readers. It blends concepts and findings with mental health implications of culture. Culture as composed of values, norms, beliefs, lifestyles, or a general way of life with a group of people with implications for mental health has also been described in detail.

Understanding the dynamic interplay of cultural forces acting on an individual can throw a light on knowing how people can cope with psychological changes.

Spirituality and well-being section encompasses the themes related to inner awareness and personal integration which can improve the wellness of an individual. The visions of spirituality can help a person to master wellness and overcome miseries. Indian spiritual traditions can act as a huge support to avoid harmful effects on mental health.

In this section on suffering and healing, the connections between cultural, subjective experiences, and well-being are explained. Buddhism perspective, in particular the method of mindfulness, is found to be useful in the healing.

Finally, this chapter presents a brief overview of the concepts and reciprocal relations of stress, ecology, work–life balance, mental health, and well-being. It also deals with the ideas of mental health and well-being in terms of examining them in detail in separate chapters. By consolidating both theories of mental health and well-being, research and critical ideas can offer a novel perspective to understand these subjects.

This book on mental health and well-being attempts to address the issues and perspectives pertaining to mental health and well-being. The chapters and pages of this book are intended to imparting conceptual and empirical explanations of the relevant knowledge and insights of this field.

Its pages are full of valuable information about interconnection of mental health and well-being from the horizons of eastern and Western knowledge systems. Most significant accounts of the intellectual, spiritual, ecological, and cultural domains have been provided in a novel way, likely to be useful to readers and especially to those intelligible minds desirous of insightful connections. It remains distinctive to point out that the very nature of mental health is affected by diversities of ecology, culture, oriental and accidental perspectives of suffering, and healing and spirituality factors. It appears to me that it is high time that all thoughtful academicians and researchers should reconsider their position to analyse the issue of mental health merely from DSM and ICD perspectives and refocus their attention from an alternative perspective.

A common philosophical creed had prevailed in India long before the crystallization of rationalistic inquiry into separate systems and categories. Various Indian philosophical schools of *Vedanta*, *Upanishads*, *Nyay, Vaisheshika, Samkhaya*, Yoga, *Purava-mimansa, Vedanta*, Jainism. The *Charvaka Bhagavad Gita* tends to provide a more synthetic approach for a comprehensive vision. It is with the synthetic vision of Indian philosophy that higher vision of human knowledge, its complexities, and difficulties can be resolved, and a transfer from *avidya* (ignorance) to *vidya* (knowledge) of human beings can be achieved.

Think Box

Reflect upon the Indian perspectives of understanding mental health. How is it similar/different from the Western notions of mental health and mental illness?

Chapter 1 Introduction to Mental Health and Well-being

Key points:

1. Trephining is considered to be one of the earliest surgical method.
2. Hippocrates believed that mental illness was an organic illness, not caused by demons.
3. Exorcism occurs when a demon is commanded by a priest in the name of God to stop his activity within a person.
4. Johann Weyer is recognized as the first physician to specialize in the treatment of melancholy.
5. The response of the society to mental illness is categorized in three phases in time: Renaissance phase, Classical phase, and Modern age.
6. Stigma, labelling, and prejudice are factors deterring mentally ill patients from seeking treatment.
7. The origin of stress maybe biogenic, psychogenic, or contextual or a combination of all.
8. Work–life balance equilibrium is supported by the concepts of happiness and achievement.
9. According to Buddhism, there are four unavoidable sufferings: birth, old age, sickness, and death.
10. The tendency to view one's group and its cultural expectations or rights to be superior to others is called Ethnocentrism.

Key Words:

Trephining, Exorcism, Melancholy, Stigma, Taboo, Anthropocene, Eudaimonic, Cultural pluralism, Transcendent, Mechanical solidarity

References

Almeida-Filho, N., Mari, J., Coutinho, E., França, J. F., Fernandes, J., Andreoli, S. B., & Brussello, E. D. (1997). Brazilian multicentric study of psychiatric morbidity. Methodological features and prevalence estimates. *The British Journal Of Psychiatry: The Journal of Mental Science*, *171*, 524–529.

Baglio, M. (2010). *The rite: The making of a modern exorcist*. Image Books/Double Day.

Cavanaugh, R. (2015). From demons to doctors. *History Today Ltd*, *65*(4), 44–45.

Faria, M. (2013). Violence, mental illness and the brain – A brief history of psychosurgery: Part 1: From trephination to lobotomy. *Surgical Neurology International*, *4*(49).

Foucault, M. (2009). *History of madness*. Routledge.

Freud, S. (1900). The interpretation of dreams. In J. Strachey (Ed.), *The standard edition of the complete works of Sigmund Freud* (Vols. 4 and 5). Hogarth Press.

Haque, A. (2004). Psychology from Islamic perspective: Contributions of early Muslim scholars and challenges to contemporary Muslim psychologists. *Journal of Religion and Health*, *43*, 357–377.

Hollander, B. (2015). *Nervous disorders of women (psychology rituals)*. Routledge.

India State-Level Disease Burden Initiative Mental Disorders Collaborators (2020). The burden of mental disorders across the states of India: The Global Burden of Disease Study 1990–2017. *The Lancet. Psychiatry*, *7*(2), 148–161. https://doi.org/10.1016/S2215-0366(19)30475-4

Institute for Health Metric and Evaluation (2017). *Global burden of disease study*. The LANCET (W.H.O.).

Khetan, P. P. (2008). *The Bhagvad Gita*, Chapter 2, verse 47 (pp. 59–60). Sri Aurobindo Divine Life Trust Jhunjhnu. ISBN: 81-865 10-03-6.

Kleisiaris, C. F., Sfakianakis, C., & Papathanasious, I. V. (2014). Health care practices in Ancient Greece, The Hippocratic ideal. *Journal of Medical Ethics and History of Medicine*, *7*, 6.

Mahdi, M., Gutas, D., Abed, S. B. et al. (1987). *Avicena encyclopedia Ironica* (Vol. 3). Routledge and Kegan Paul.

National Mental Health Survey of India (2015–16). *National mental health survey of India*. National Institute of Mental Health and Neurosciences Bengaluru and Ministry of Health & Family Welfare. Government of India.

Nizamie, H. S., & Goyal, N. (2010, January). History of psychiatry in India. *Indian Journal of Psychiatry*, *52*.

Porter, R. (2002). *Madness: A brief history*. Oxford University Press.

Regier, D. A., Boyd, J. H., Burke, J. D., Jr, Rae, D. S., Myers, J. K., Kramer, M., Robins, L. N., George, L. K., Karno, M., & Locke, B. Z. (1988). One-month prevalence of mental disorders in the United States. Based on five epidemiologic catchment area sites. *Archives of General Psychiatry*, *45*(11), 977–986. https://doi.org/10.1001/archpsyc.1988.01800350011002

World Health Organization's Mental Health Gap Action Programme (2008). *MhGAP: Mental health gap action programme – scaling up care for mental, neurological, and substance use disorders*. World Health Organization.

2 Stress and Coping

Learning Objectives

After reading this chapter, you will be able to understand:

- Modernity, technology, capitalism, and stress.
- Mass-media and stress
- Coping with stress
- Indian perspectives of coping

Introduction

Stress is a widespread phenomenon which can have devastating consequences for individuals and the society. The origin of the term 'stress' lies in physics rather than psychology. The concept of stress has undergone several transitions from physiological, to psychological condition, to work and environment conditions, and, finally, to a most prevalent socio-cultural phenomenon.

Initial researches in the field of psychology emphasized that stress is developed through a transition between individual factors and environmental factors. American psychologist Richard Lazarus defined stress as a mismatch of the perceived demands of a situation and the individual's assessment of his or her resources to deal with these demands (Lazarus, 1966).

The current and elaborate definition of stress is 'a particular relationship between the person and the environment that is appraised by the person as taking or exceeding his or her resources and endangering his or her well-being' (Lazarus & Folkman, 1984, p. 9). We need to examine the role of factors, and they should include individual cognitive factors focusing on personality traits influences, situational aspects, contextual factors, historical factors, and social, cultural factors. History, furthermore, provides an understanding of why certain ideas may be more accepted at one time than another and thereby addresses the influence of cultural factors on the precisions of knowledge about stress (Cooper & Dew, 2004). The individualistic stress model places the causes of stress and responsibility to cope with

DOI: 10.4324/9781003350651-2

stress on the individual, whereas distributed theory of stress attributes more importance to discussion and cultural and contextual factors. The term stress was identified by words such as 'shellshock' and 'nerve shocks' during earlier times. In 1915, D. Forsyth's article about stress conditions titled 'Functional never disease and the shock of battle. A study of the so called traumatic neurosis arising in connection to the war' appeared describing symptoms of war experiences during World War I (Forsyth, 1915). In 1916, the term 'war neurosis' began to appear in research (Eden, 1916), which resembled the stress concepts of modern times.

Hans Seleye used the term 'stress' in 1936 and defined it as being the sum of all nonspecifically induced changes in a biological system (Viner, 1999). Seleye named the non-specific sign of bodily damage 'general adaptation syndrome' and used 'stress' to describe the state of an organism in adaptation and responding to the environment. Lazarus became one of the pioneers of stress research with his studies. The effects of psychological stress upon performance (Lazarus & Ericksen, 1952) and 'Effects of failure stress upon skill performance (Lazarus & Eriksen, 1952) another landmark contribution in the field of stress was the book 'Men Under Stress' (Grinker & Spielgel, 1945).

Lazarus began theorizing about his appraisal concept and identified the kinds of appraising as being primary and secondary. Primary appraisal addresses the significance of the encounter if is it threatening or beneficial towards a person's well-being. Secondary appraisal refers to the process that focuses on evaluating the coping options (Lazarus & Folkman, 1984).

Stress as a neurological condition is concerned with disturbances in the nervous system, and as a physiological condition it is related to physiological change as a result of evolutionary pressures resulting into fight or height responses.

Stress as a result of interactions between cognitive processes focuses more upon appraisal aspects. In the later years of stress-related research, Lazarus shifted his focus from stress to its coping processes.

Coping is the ability and efforts of an individual to handle a difficult situation in his/her environment and minimize its harmful effects.

The transition of people from agrarian to industrial society used to more complex, mechanical, and repetitive work led to the dominance of stress at the workplace. The transition from mechanical to automation and computer model age led to the growth of stress at individual and organizational levels.

New skills demanded by modern-day vertical organizations also required more flexibility traits to adjust and ability to react to changes with short notice. Digital stress causes psychological ill-health effects owing to the vast expansion of Internet-mediated communication in personal and professional lives. Communication load results from social media messages as well as from Internet multitasking. Perceived social pressure and the fear of missing out on information and social interaction are key features of media-mediated communication. The impact of social media on the mental health of adolescents and youth has become a priority both at national and international levels. Techno stress is created by an excessive use of technology by role conflict and role overload. Challenges arising from an excessive use of digital platforms engagements are blurring of boundaries between family life and professional life. Media-mediated activities have no limitation of time and place, and they have given rise to blurred boundaries between formal and informal life activities.

Cultural Patterning of Stress

Stress or suffering is ubiquitous, and at some point of time all human race suffers. At some occasions, it seems to be an individual-centric phenomenon, but in reality it has several others dimensions. Culture can affect the stress and the process of coping because of its appraisal in a given context and choice of strategy an individual may adopt in a given cultural context. Cultural aspects affect both situational demands and individual resources which in turn can affect the appraisal of stress. Certain stressful events are normative which majority of the people in a particular culture might experience such as onset of puberty or retirement after job.

For example qualifying in civil service examinations or securing very high percentage of marks in the board examinations shows academic brilliance among the students in Indian context. Though a selective number of students who make it to civil services and secure high percentage are satisfied, but a large majority of them experience a culturally mandated stress life situation to prove their worth. The number of students appearing for NEET exams entrance in India are more than a million, but only very less percentage of them finally qualify for admission. The IIT-JEE is a dream destination for majority of students with an engineering bent of mind in India. In 2014, 13.6 lakhs students sat for the IIT-JEE exams, and only 9,784 seats were available in the IITs put together. The acceptance rate (5.8%) at Harvard is among the lowest in US universities, and is ironically eight times easier to get into them. IITs though have different criteria for admission.

Kota city in Rajasthan is considered as a famous place for providing quality coaching for getting through entrance examinations of various technical courses to students, and they come from all over India to here to pursue their educational dreams. The enormous amount of parental and societal pressure leads them to anxiety and depression. In extreme situations, unrealistic expectations of parents and teachers have also driven few of them to commit suicide in the past. Nowhere in the world does one find coaching for entrance examination to technical courses having such high stakes in a student's admission as it is in India.

Cultural psychology framework is the ontological view on socio-genesis, the view that the human mind is social because of emergence of mind in a social context.

Depending on personal constitution, individuals internalize cultural suggestions and find some form of translation in the mind of these cultural, tools, signs and modes of interaction (Valsiner, 1998, 2007).

Culture is considered to be a set of semiotic and material resources characterized by a dialogical interaction between individual and resources in the environment, and people's discourses shape an individual's interpretations of the world. One of the basic assumptions in the dialogical perspective is that a person organizes inner dialogues guided by the social world (Markova, 2006; Valsiner, 1998). Hermans employs the concept of the dialogical self, which he describes as 'a dynamic multiplicity of I-positions in the landscape of the mind intertwined as this mind is with the minds of other people' (Hermans, 2001, p. 243).

The concept of distributed cognition is different from the traditional approach of cognition limiting it into the head of individuals. The role of social, cultural, and technological factors suggests the importance of ecological surroundings on cognition.

Hutchins (1995) argues that 'human cognition is not just inference by culture and society, but that it is in a very fundamental sense a cultural and social process' (p. xiv) cultural psychology perspective of stress of an individual one must take into account the embeddedness of contexts, local discourses into consideration.

Stress is considered to be a dialogical phenomenon based on people making sense of the world with others and interpretation of events.

Stress: A Socially Embedded Model

Social embeddedness of stress can be explained with the other people's experiences and interpretations of the world through an exchange of signs.

Positive construct meanings range from dialogism perspective through a field of opposites. The coping process is also distributed among members of a social group. From the semiotics perspective, the appraisal and coping process is dialogical in nature mediated through the use of language in social interactions. As Linell underlines, 'distributed cognitions is typically understood a distributed along the extended loop of body-drain systems, artifacts semiotic resources and the material world but to this list we should add 'the other and her actions and utterances' (Linell, 2009, p. 146).

It is significant to mention that the conceptualization of stress as a product of individuals versus environment is contrasted in social perspective emphasizing the interdependent interaction with others.

The role of others gets a central place, and it has implications for the coping mechanisms.

Coping for stress like other psychological processes is a normative process with the individual implicitly or explicitly comparing oneself with other.

The process of coping is always relative to social norms allowing persons to assess whether one's coping capabilities are mostly result of their social positioning generally ignored by individualistic framework.

The concept of extended mind used by Clark and Chalmers (1998) is a version of 'active externalism' which states that significant parts of what constitutes mental functioning exist outside the skill of the individual.

There is a need to comprehend the realty of stress from a more dynamic perspective, and cognition is a multilayered process of problem-solving interpreting and judging. Mechanic (1974) argued that the efficacy of an individual's coping mechanism is largely determined how well their culture provides a range of coping resources and transmits coping skills. The formal social and cultural institutions specialized for providing means of conflict solution influence coping strategies adopted by the individuals. There are also rituals and some forms of ritualized advice that may be given by religious counsellors for full-counselling service which can suggest culturally appropriate roles for coping.

People may have to perform different social roles in their life journey which may give rise to stressors. Certain life events can cause stress that alters the role of an individual, possibly citing a chronic type of stressor (Pearlin, 1991). Roles considered to be significant in one's life journey include education, occupation, parenthood, marriage, family, and economy. The theoretical perspective of viewing roles as contexts calls attention to status which exists not only as an attribute to the individuals but also can be conceptualized as part of contextual social inequality' as existing across 'multiple layers of social hierarchy' (Aneshensel, 2010, p. 35).

Role Strain

Role strain theory suggests that society puts pressure on individuals to achieve socially desirable goals despite lacking the means to do so.

Robert K. Merton's (1938) theory known as strain theory explained that when individuals are faced with a gap between their goals and their current status, strain occurs. Merton outlines five different ways people may respond when faced with strain (Merton, 1938).

(i) Conformity – pursuing socio-cultural goals that are socially approved ('hopeful poor').
(ii) Innovation using acceptance of social goals but trying different and unconventional ways to achieve them ('surviving poor').
(iii) Ritualism – Using the same social, approved means to achieve less elusive goals ('passive poor').
(iv) Retreatism – to reject enter the cultural goals and means to obtain it then find a way to escape it ('Retreating poor')
(v) Rebellion to reject cultural goals and the prescribed means to achieve them, then work towards replacing both of them ('resisting poor').

The strain is a result of a gap in the expectations and means for their fulfilment. These gaps in expectations and their fulfilment can take place in personal domain, social domains, relational domains, professional domains, or a combination of domains. The gaps exists expectations, aspirations, or a conflict between two equally relevant values, perceived sense of deprivation and lack of coping resources at individual and social level. Strain theory of suicide suggests that suicide is usually preceded by prolonged psychological strain (Merton, 1938).

Pearlin (1983) identified six types of role strains which are experienced in participation of social roles.

(i) Problems between an individual and the nature of a role task: For example a role assigned by others even though related to one's work may appear as an overload if not self-chosen.
(ii) Interpersonal conflict: This type of strain occurs due to disagreements resulting into differences while working with other people.
(iii) Role captivity: Such type of strain occurs when a person experiences discrepancy between his/her current role and a desired goal.
(iv) The loss and gain of roles that demand adaptation: such type of strain is experienced when people lack pre-socialization for new roles suddenly coming their way. Becoming a patient, sudden divorce, or involuntary job loss are some of the examples related to this concept.
(v) Role restructuring: Sudden change of roles and responsibilities brings status and privilege changes which may result in strain.
(vi) Multiple roles and intrapersonal conflict: It is most commonly observed that participation in multiple roles may create strains as some of the demands may be conflicting with each other.

The Stress of Mastery Delusion

Mastery refers to the individual perceptions of ability to handle stress (Pearlin & Bierman, 2013). A positive correlation between mastery as a resource and socio-economic status is suggested with the resources in this field.

A high socio-economic status is also associated with higher status (educational and occupation) which contributes to a sense of self-confidence. A sense of mastery can reduce the impact and threat caused by strain with a perceived sense of higher self-efficacy and perceived social support. Beyond a moderate point, the sense of mastery can acquire the form of delusion. Having too much of confidence and trying things beyond the scope of one's abilities can result into deleterious effects.

Lack of Social Diversity Appreciation

We live in a world populated by people and groups who are different from us. Diversity is the presence of difference and most commonly referred to social difference. Most important aspects of diversity include topics of gender diversity race, diversity, disability, religion, caste, social class, age, and sexual orientation.

Psychologists and demographers show a common interest in social categories also used for describing people. Mere social categorization into groups is sufficient to produce discrimination as people favour their own groups and discriminate others. Stereotypic generalizations can constrain the emergence of low status groups. Dominant groups in the society achieve legitimacy of their superiority and coercion by ideological means of legitimacy and inducing a state of false consciousness among such ordinated groups.

In past few decades, lot of violence relating to gender, caste, religion, and race has taken place which is closely associated with dominance attitude, beliefs, and behaviour of the dominant class.

There are psychological outcomes of fear, anxiety, anguish, humiliation, or diminished self-esteem by the members of victimized groups.

Multiculturalism is the name ascribed to belief or ideas that promote the recognition, appreciation, celebration, and preservation of social difference. A patchwork quilt metaphor is used by educators to teach diversity concepts for appreciating multiculturalism.

In the spirit of the metaphor and values surrounding multiculturalism, the diversity of quilt preserves the uniqueness of social and cultural groups for a superordinate purpose.

The melting pot ideal involves the acceptance of other's differences, especially those that relate to distinct social category are blended into a single social and cultural unity.

Social justice can be preserved when all groups in a society are afforded equal rights, and spirits are not unfairly constrained by prejudice and discrimination.

Technology, Modernity, and Well-being

Before the advent of industrialization, the nature of societies was largely agrarian with dependence on man-made things.

The term 'collective consciousness' was used to refer to people's face-to-face interaction during this era.

The lifestyles of people were based upon need-based exchanges of items with a strong sense of social bonding and sharing of common social norms. The introduction of technology-mediated assembly lines led to the experiences of alienation among the working class.

Advancement of technologies and the concept of eugenics led to the ideologization of science and technology as a symbol of national dignity and achievements.

The rapid pace of technological advancements contributed to the creation of more needs and more new technology which eventually resulted into mass alienation. Theoretical framework of dialectical materialism meant constant social tensions and conflicts due to differences in distribution of income wealth, power, prestige, and control resulting from unequal control over the means of production.

Think Box

Is technology has resulted into social alienation?

Profit-making attitude became the dominant philosophy of capitalism which resulted in self-centeredness and accumulation of power and wealth in the hands of a few people. Poverty of the masses was the consequence of this materialistic philosophy. Francis Bacon succinctly put it as 'science abandons its search for truth and turns to the search for power'. Fordism is considered to be the landmark of the models of economic expansion and technological progress. Based on mass production, post Fordism era brought standardization methods of production, and economics of scale were replaced with organizations and economies of scope. Mass production and assembly lines involved repetitive work, night shifts, unhygienic working conditions which adversely affected the well-being of the workers' mass production. Technology-mediated activities contributed to the feelings of isolation, lack of involvement, and poor health among the factory workers.

Technology acquired the space for interaction, compassion, and companions, which robbed humans of their natural abilities and capacities.

The concept of techno stress was introduced by Bord (1984) who defined it as 'a madness diseases of adaptation caused by an inability to cope with the new computer technologies in a healthy manner'. It manifests itself in two distinct and related ways in the struggle to accept computer technology and in the more specialized form of over-identification with computer technology. As a result he is either struggling to accept computer technology or being over identified with computer technology.

Techno stress is caused by various factors of techno-overload, techno-invasion, techno-complexity, and techno-uncertainty.

Ergonomics is the discipline of designing tools and work environments to optimize performance and behaviours. Ergonomics aims to minimize the stressful effects of machines on human beings (Bord, 1984).

In the technological structure, man and machines are interchangeable, and both are subject to an abstract calculation of their quantifiable value.

Workers in the factories are equated with commodities as they move in a material world increasingly made up of commodities. This occurs because workers own nothing but labour to sell and thus can be bought.

Digital Technologies and Human Well-being

Our lives have become immersed in technology. Most of our activities, our communication, leisure, and entertainment are online, and for the majority of the people, mobile phones have become an integral part of their existence. The Internet has become a valuable learning resource, and its excess usage interferes with personal and social well-being, also associated with a range of psycho-social difficulties.

Neuroscience has become an effective source of insight into understanding how we can interact with technology.

Valkenburg and Peter identified three key aspects of psycho-social development including identity, intimacy, and sexuality which can be influenced by online communication (Valkenburg et al., 2005).

Teenagers are one of the most avid users of online communication, and its advantages and disadvantages are related to usage durations and quality of interaction. In 2003, Green Bavelier studied visual processing skills of gamers as compared with non-gamers and found that playing videogames was associated with enhanced visual attention capacity, superior allocation of spatial attention over the visual field, and improved temporal processing of visual information (i.e. gamers were less likely to suffer 'bottlenecks' of 'attention' when many events occurred in quick successions).

Influence of Social Media

The World Health Organization (WHO, 2017) reported that 10.20% of children and adolescents worldwide experience mental health problems. It is estimated that 50% of all mental disorders are established by the age of 14 and 75% by the age of 18 (Kessler et al., 2007; Kim-Cohen et al., 2003).

The most prevalent disorders in children and adolescents have been generalized as anxiety disorders and depression, respectively, in the past few years.

The prevalence of anxiety and depression has increased in the past few years in young people and adolescents. The rising incidence of mental health problems is influenced by more information sharing in the digital age, lack of mental health awareness initiatives, and the development of complex relations in the society.

The term 'social media' refers to the various internet-based networks that enable users to interact with others, verbally or visually (Carr & Hayes, 2015).

Multitasking is a very common thing for adolescents and youth, which affects the psychological well-being depending upon its content and prolonged usage durations. The factors of social isolation, loneliness, and a lack of interest in social activities contribute to the distress among the users of social media directly and indirectly.

Excess use of social media on a regular basis may contribute to distress and anxiety problems among the users.

Adolescents are highly attracted towards media gadgets and media influences. In the contemporary times, adolescents and the youth use Internet which affects all areas of their development which includes behavioural, social, cognitive, and creative dimensions. Social media platforms have influenced the majority of relationships with family, peers, and teachers to a large extent.

Prolonged stress may be used to the development of mental health problems. Weinstein et al. (2016) identified two types of digital stresses. The first type of stressors involve one or more of the following: mental and harassing personal attacks, public sharing and limitation and impersonation. The second, type two stressors are connected to use and/or are relational in nature. In response to the research question asking what digital stressors are over the line, Weinstein et al. (2016) indicated that vulnerability increases when digital tools are used for type 2 scenarios that promote connection and intimacy. There is always possibility and potential for digital stress to occur due to overexposure and unintended consequences.

In a study, Cingel and Krcmar (2014) revealed results that show Facebook use as positively related to behavioural rehearsal which is related to imaginary audience ideation. They also posited a Compare–Think–Act trilogy, which has adolescents comparing their behaviours to that of others, thinking of ways to achieve a desired behavioural change to appear like others, and acting in a way that achieves the desired outcomes (Cingel & Krcmar, 2014).

Think Box

1. Has social media become the largest contributor of stress?
2. Being together but alone. Discuss this statement in the light of social media.

Turkle (2015) found that youth navigate to the digital world to experiment with identify work. 'The ability to understand how navigate context, audience and identity intersects is one of the central challenges people face in learning how to navigate social media' (Boyd, 2014). The turbulent activities of the teenage phase can get amplified through interaction on social media platforms.

Defined as 'Performative, interpersonal conflict that takes place in front of an active, engaged audience, often a social media', teen drama 'does not automatically position anyone as either a target or abuser' (Boyd, 2014). Turkle (2015) reflected: 'From the early days, I saw that computer offers the illusion of companionship without demands of friendship and then, as the programs got really, good, the illusion of companionship without the demands of intimacy' (p. 7).

Collier (2014) cautioned sheltering teens from online activity and discussed about juvenoia, a term coined to describe excessive fear over society's progress and the resultant social influence.

It is true that social media devices and activities have had their impact on the range of intrapersonal and interpersonal experiences at individual and societal levels. There are variety of mediating factors, such as parental influence, personality traits, and social and cultural influences which can mitigate the negative influences of social media upon its users.

Social media platforms pose a diversity of opportunities and challenges, which is very complex. Social media offers a strong relational platform which is interconnected to the emotional and educational development, and its handling pattern may result in adaptive or maladaptive behavioural consequences for its users. Cyber culture can be characterized as a culture that has emerged from the use of computer networks for communication entertainment and business. Cyber stalking, cyber bullying, and cyber victimization have increased rapidly in Indian context in past few years. A vast majority of Internet users experience some form of a cyber victimization from peers and siblings in the form of emotional bullying, sexual misconduct or abuse, and non-contact sexual victimization or child pornography.

The Internet is a space in which criminal activities may take diverse forms without the physical presence of its actors and which benefits from the timelessness, the possibility of anonymity, and the absence of a restricted space. The activities of cybercrime can adversely affect the emotional and social development of individuals with implications of stress and mental health. The risk exposure to sexually explicit material and inappropriate content at early age may result into long-term problems in the later stages. The intersection of some disadvantaged conditions (poverty, lower socio-economic status, lack of awareness) and other demographic characteristics may enhance the risk of cumulative victimization in cyberspace. There are other risk factors associated with cybercrime which may consist of situational factors of vulnerability, sharing of personal information, frequency of virtual interaction, and surfing without parental protection, which may add to the vulnerability of offender–victim cycle.

The objective factors causing the risk of cybercrime explanations are still at an embryonic stage due to limited empirical evidences available in the field. The risky lifestyles, including the practice of crime based on computer misuse (e.g. hacking), crime against people (e.g. cyberstalking, cyberbullying), and the association with deviant cyber peers have been considered important risk factors for the increased experiences of cybercrime (Bossler et al., 2012).

The adolescent personality dispositions and suffering resulting from problems of depression, isolation, and parental rejection are more likely to face online risky behaviours. In particular, low self-confidence and self-esteem and poor social competence pose a greater vulnerability for adolescent manipulation by the cyber aggressors.

There is a no straight cause and effect relationship of cyber-crime taking place in the digital space, and inevitable exposure to digital territory requires more elaborate research evidence for arriving at a better understanding of this issue.

A multidisciplinary approach involving psychology, sociology criminology, and demographic characteristic analysis may prove crucial in understanding of the complex dynamics of cybercrime.

The subject of Internet exposure and cybercrime against adolescents has posed a moral dilemma regarding the usage of technology by the young generation, and the use of Internet as huge resource of stress at intergenerational level is undeniable (Bossler & Holt, 2009).

Capitalism and Stress

The term anxiety is used when threat is not imminent, and fear is a central theme of suffering and distress. Capitalism is about enjoyment of commodities, ostentation consumption, wealth accumulation, profit maximization, and celebrity life. The suffering that intolerable debt levels impose on people, the exit of well-functioning public institutions by private, and deprivation of local communities of poor children lead to a vicious cycle of poverty and suffering.

Klein explained the cynical economic exploitation by the capitalists caused by natural catastrophes and political upheavals by so-called 'disaster capitalism' with deleterious economic and personal consequences for the indigenous communities. It is well known that the Great Depression of 1929 witnessed many suicides on the part of the people unable to cope with the difficulties caused due to the economic hardship.

In recent times, suicides have again become a barometer for the psychological ill effects of financial and economic hardship being faced by farmers, students, and labourers.

In order to highlight the link between capitalism and suffering under normal conditions, the views of Ian Parker, a practicing Lacanian psychoanalyst, are more apt, who associate suffering under capitalism with obsessional neurosis (Parker, 2011, p. 42) and writes 'Those who suffer in obsessional mode under capitalism are subjects who buy into the separation of intellectual and manual labour, the separation of thinking from being and live out the predicament of a puzzle about the nature of being as if false consciousness really did operate only at the level of the individual. Lacan argues that the question that haunts the obsessional neurotic concern being, existence their right to exist and whether they are alive or dead . . . . The obsessions are repetitive ideas manifested in a series of actions from which the subject seems unable to escape. Even though this eventually may result in suffering that is too much to bear, enough to bring someone to ask for help, it is still stubbornly tied to administrative strategies that contain an unbearable surplus of satisfaction – 'jouissance' is name for this excess – within the domain of the pleasure principle. The attributes of obsessional neurosis are recognizable in repetitive actions, in eradicable guilt uncertainty and anxiety, which are the manners which people show in the contemporary capitalist society. The other important aspects of alienation, powerlessness, resentment, and exploitation are the fundamental textures of capitalism where manifested rationality of production and consumption turns into irrationality which breaks the trust between subjects and market, and subjects become products of capitalism. In *The Shock doctrine: The Rise of Disaster Capitalism* by

Naomi Klein, The Times, October 12, 2007 described about the latest incarnation of the capitalist juggernaut as driven by the ideological imperative, to privatize every aspect of an economy (local or national) while communities or nations are in a state of disoriented shock in the wake of a collective natural or political trauma.

In her incisive book *Tyranny of Choice,* Renata Salecl (2010) probes what she calls the 'tyranny of choice' and argues that ours is a capitalistic society thriving on a bewildering array of things, items, products, services, even short-term sex partners, or companies manifested as giving economic and social freedom, but in reality all of it comes at a price. Salecl wrote (2010, pp. 8–9).

> In today's society, which glorifies choice and the idea that choice is always is people's interests, the problem is not just the scale of choice available but the manner in which choice is represented. Life choices are described in same terms as consumer choices: We set out to find the right life as we would find the right kind of wallpaper or hair conditioners. Today's advice culture presents the search for a spouse as not all that different from the search for a car. The issue of choice has been a concerns primarily of the middle classes in the developing world yet even in poor countries may have been troubled by the contradictions interest in the ideology of choice supposedly now free to make whatever they want out of their lives, in reality they live in an ideal world and as though the choices they make are reversible; while the reality is that their economic circumstances prevent them from having much freedom of choice at all and that one wrong decision can have disastrous consequences.

The ideology of choice perpetuated by capitalism tends to ensure capitalism hegemony by inculcating a collective mindset oriented according to its precepts. Through the emergence of advice culture, an individual moves from initial necessity to choose the negation of one's choice and desire by replacing with other's desire leading to a mounting pressure of insecurity and anxiety on oneself, often leading to depression. Salecl (2010, p. 15) argued that people, when confronted with a range of alternatives, fall back on either a random choice owing to volitional paralysis or shifting to the basal option triggered by an 'automatic' awareness of the most advertised production which can further increase anxiety and feelings of inadequacy.

Adaptation to capitalist society norms requires conforming to the demands of market-oriented dictates of consumption. The conflicts for identity in a market-based society are determined by how we are related to our bodies, our partners, our colleagues, and family – in short, to our identities.

These are growing signs of people realizing that psychic pathologies reflect social censure on the basis of accepted social norms of any given time (Focault, 1980, *History of Sexuality*). It is important to mention that illness paradigms suggested by DSM are lopsided, and they fall short of incorporating social and cultural economic aspects of illness. In the year 2000, the Harvard review of psychiatry referred to social phobia as being the third most frequent psychiatric disorder after depression and alcoholism. The problems related to inequality of incomes in a society lead to trust deficit, more fear, and less participation in the community life, which also contribute to the health of the population. According to Silvia Federici, throughout its history, capitalism has transformed our bodies into work machines which is being manifested in the social and individual pathologies, the resistance, the refusals, and search for new anthropological paradigm (Federici, 2013, p. 3). It is argued that disciplines like philosophy and psychology have contributed to the crises faced by capitalism, and a need for reconstructed psychology is the need of the time if it wishes to separate its history of complicity and collaborations with power (Federici, 2013, p. 3).

Contemporary capitalistic milieu transforms the labour power into 'mechanization of body', ignoring the disgust of the regimentation of their minds and bodies by industrial labour.

Federici (2013, p. 7) notes:

> Indeed the abstraction and regimentation of labor has reached today its completion and so has its own sense of alienation and desocialization. What levels of stress this situation is producing in our lives can be measured by massification of mental diseases panic, anxiety, fear, attention deficit, the escalating consumption of drugs from prozac to viagra. Fear and anxiety are only one aspect of the terror that today is employed to suffocate the growing revolt against the global work machine. Equally important has been the militarization of everyday life now an international trend preceding September 11.

In contemporary times, there are myriads of reasons for emergence of stress unregulated by work, subject to the identity destructive market and people are experiencing gestation of a new imaginary from the homogenizing tendency of capitalist globalization. This eco-destructive exploitation model of consumerist capitalism and ongoing automation has led to dehumanization of human behaviour. People in the modern capitalistic era are becoming more isolated from real social and political sphere, producing more stress and anxiety. There is plenty of evidence in the capitalistic era in the form of CMI, credit, cards, home loans, educational loans, car loans promoting individualism which may result in suffering in the form of cluster of interrelated psychic phenomena – such as anxiety, self-doubt, depression, and debilitating uncertainty inseparable from the culture of choice.

Darian Leader (2008, pp. 1–2) highlights the negative side of modern individualism, where each of us is taken to be an isolated agent, cut off from others and driven by competition for goods and services in the market-place rather than by community and shared effort.

People in general are getting disconnected or less connected with rituals of communal ties and moving towards having 'quick-fix solutions' approach in life.

Coping With Stress and Indian Perspectives of Coping

Coping With Stress

The word 'cope' is derived from the Latin word 'Colpus' meaning 'to after' and, as defined in the Webster's dictionary, is usually used in the psychological paradigm 'overcome problems and difficulties'. Psychoanalytic theory describes coping as a defence mechanism for protecting individuals. Psychoanalysts describe defence mechanisms of introjections, reaction formation, regression sublimation, denial, intellectualization, and others used for protection from both internal and external threats. Individuals also use adaptations and mastery to overcome anxiety. Lazarus and Folkman in (1984) the book *Stress, Appraisal, and Coping* is an application of thought processes and behavioral efforts to compact demands that exceed a person resources. This view of coping treats coping as opposed to personality traits, physiological response, and the mastery concepts.

Choice of a coping strategy is a dynamic process which is influenced by a variety of factors such as knowledge, skills, attitudes, and social resources.

Vulnerability and ability to cope are two sides of the same coin. There are several day-to-day practical solutions used for coping with stress which may include relaxation, breathing exercises, good nutrition, yoga, and music which can go a long way to help people manage stressful situations.

Personality and Coping

Personality is a very broad topic which encompasses partly statements about what makes everyone the same and what makes people differ from each other. There are various models and theories which explain different individuals. Human nature can be described from various perspectives, but the biological models and goal-based models are relevant in the context of stress and coping.

Biological model holds that approach and avoidance are partly guided by distinct brain areas which ultimately influence the behaviour of a person towards environmental rewards and threats. The mechanism of effortful control also guides a person to arrive at behavioural decisions.

Another approach in personality theory projects goal-directed quality of behaviour. In goal-based theories, it is important to distinguish between motivational properties aimed at moving towards goals and those aimed at staying away from threats (Carver & Scheier, 2008; Elliot, 2008; Higgins, 1996). Designed goal induces positive incentive values, and difficulty in attaining a desired goal induces a negative incentive value. Goal-based models also typically incorporate an expectancy construct: a sense of confidence or doubt that a given outcome will be attained successfully (e.g. Bandura, 1986; Carver & Scheier, 1998). Expectations of achieving or failing are considered to be important determinants of people's efforts.

The extraversion factor of five-factor theory relates to confidence, dominance, and sense of sociality. In certain research situations, extraversion is found to be useful with researches in this field indicating positive connection of extraversion and approach to temperament and neuroticism with avoidance temperament. Agreeableness factor is also considered to be helpful in coping mechanisms. Agreeable people get less angry over others' transgressions than do less agreeable people (Meier & Robinson, 2004), and this seems to defuse the possibility of aggression. People with good relationships generally maintain a higher degree of agreeableness with others.

The factors of conscientiousness and being open to experience which are fourth and fifth factors of big time factors' theory also play a positive role in the coping mechanism. Optimism is a significant contributor in the coping processes.

A particularly important distinction is there between engagement or approach coping, which is aimed at dealing with stress or on related emotions and disengagement or avoidance coping which is aimed at escaping the threat or related emotions (e.g. Moos & Schaefer, 1993; Roth & Cohen, 1986; Skinner et al., 2003).

Engagement coping is basically problem-focused coping which may involve support seeking and cognitive restructuring. Disengagement coping is mainly emotion-focused coping, which may involve attempts to escape the conditions of stress as if it does not exist. The concept of disengagement coping has been extended to include relinquishing goals that are threatened by the stressor (Carver et al., 1989).

Accommodative Coping and Meaning-Focused Coping

Accommodative coping involves attempts to adapt or adjust to the stresses. Accommodative coping involves responses of acceptance as well. Cognitive restructuring and modifying one's goals in the light of excessive threats to oneself. Meaning-focused coping is a strategy adopted by people in which they draw a positive experience of stress. This construct has roots in evidence that positive as well as negative emotions are common during stressful experiences, and people may try to find positives even during difficult times.

Proactive Coping

Some form of coping that occurs even before the emergence of stress is known as proactive coping.

Personality dimensions certainly influence the process of coping in many ways. The factors of attentional regulation, temperament, and expectancy value play a role in the coping mechanisms. There are a number of studies which establish associations between personality and coping. Relations between personality and coping were generally stronger in samples facing a high degree of stress (e.g. cancer, chronic pain, divorce) than in samples with little stress (Connor-Smith & Flachsbart, 2007). Relations of five-factor traits with emotion-focused coping also suggest the importance of distinguishing between types of emotion-focused coping (Connor-Smith & Flachsbart, 2007).

Situational versus dispositional coping

Dispositional factors of personality are also guided by situational factors in the process of coping. Response of a person at the time of stress is also influenced by the type of event, available resources, and controllability factor. Another important moderator is the time lag or the time elapsed in aggregating the responses related to the same event.

Personality Relations with Mental and Physical Health:

Meta-analyses related to the link between personality and psychological consequences show strong linkages. Neuroticism is linked to greater risk for suicide ideation, attempts, and completion (Brezo et al., 2006). Pessimism is related to lower levels of subjective well-being across many studies (Carver et al., 2009). Extraversion is strongly associated with measures of well-being, explaining up to 19% of variance in positive mood (Steel et al., 2008). Extraversion is negatively associated with suicidality (Brezo et al., 2006) and with clinical symptoms in general, particularly symptoms of mood, anxiety, and eating disorders. Several studies indicate a greater longevity with optimism and conscientiousness. Strong links between personality factors and coping outcomes can be reasonably assumed on the basis of several researches. It is also important to focus the attention of researchers to models of personality other than big five factors.

Think Box

1. How do traits interact in determining coping responses?
2. What are fundamental distinctions between engagement coping and disengagement coping?
3. Relations between personality traits coping is moderated by other varieties of age, time, severity. Discuss.

Developmental Conceptualizations of Coping

Coping is considered to have significant links with other developing subsystems such as language and culture. Coping is a conscious and volitional effort to regulate emotion, cognition, and behaviour, and it is influenced by a variety of developmental factors. Kopp (1989), a pioneer in the work on the development of emotion regulation (ER), argues that 'Emotion regulation is a term used to characterize the processes and characteristics involved in coping with heightened levels of positive and negative emotions' (p. 343).

Functionalist theorists place central importance on emotion in coping. Emotion is considered integral to all phases of the coping process including detection, appraisal, and co-ordinating responses.

Dual process models of coping:

The concept of emotional regulation describes two important aspects – one describing the target to be regulated such as emotional impulse and other describing the processes used to regulate it. In work on emotion there are referred to as emotion and emotion regulation (Cole et al., 2004) in work on temperament 'reactivity' and 'regulation' (Rothbart et al., 1994) in work on will power, the 'hot' emotional and the 'cool' cognitive systems (Metcalfe & Mischel, 1999) in work on motivations 'intrinsic' and 'extrinsic' motivation [Deci & Ryan, 1985].

Reactions and responses from emotional systems are also described as 'go' responses requiring quick readiness to respond to a variety of situations such as threat or anger.

Dual process model of Compas and Colleagues (1997, 1999) distinguishes between involuntary stress responses, which describe immediate and automatic reactions to stressful situations, and coping, which refers to 'regulatory efforts that are volitionally and intentionally enacted specifically in response to stress' (Compas et al., 2001, p. 89). There are several coping categories which have emerged from research on coping, and important among them include problem solving, support seeking, resilience adaptation, and competence. Coping responses are also categorized as higher-order categories of coping and lower-order categories of coping.

Skinner et al. (2003) identified a smaller number of families of coping with each family of higher-order consisting of a few lower-order ways of coping. Higher-order families of coping include responses of problem-solving, support-seeking, escape, distraction, cognitive restructuring, and so on. It is interesting to point out that these families of coping are developed in nature and get more differentiated with advancing age.

Coping is also influenced by socialization processes especially children copying parents play a dominant role in the determination of stressors and children with impersonal minds which ultimately affects children's coping skills.

The research on coping suggests that better coping skills can be learned through exposure to a diversity of contents. Apart from individual processes, the role of interpersonal processes and larger social ecological contexts can help in the improvement of coping resources.

Think Box

1. How does social contexts shape the development of coping?
2. How can coping resources be promoted?

Indian Perspective of Coping

In India, family is the most important institution that has survived through ages. It is considered to be a collectivistic society in which interdependence and co-operation with family members in difficult situations are considered as duty. The joint family has always been the preferred family type in Indian culture, and three to four generations of family members co-exist through kinship bonds. Adaptation, self-sacrifice, and tolerance to the views of elders are preferred values of the Indian society. Child-rearing practices and providing a supportive environment lead to the emotional growth of children. Children are expected to listen, respect, and obey their parents, and it enhances feelings of togetherness in the family. Indian culture places a lot of importance on societal values.

As Kakar (1979) stated 'In its social implication, dharma is an inherent force in human being which holds the individual and society after together' or going a step further, force which makes 'individual and society hold each other together'. (P-6). The philosophical and spiritual elements present in Indian culture act as a support to deal with difficulties in life. The broader life cycle of an Individual is contingent on four factors: (a) desk (country, region); (b) *kala* (period of history); (c) *shrama* (work); and (d) *guna* (biomental attributes).

Transgression of *dharma* is considered to be the root cause of human suffering and conflicts. As a social being, people tend to have a strong existence with a rich network of relationships which shape one's identity. *Dukha* or suffering is an important concept in Hinduism and Buddhism, which is somewhat connected to the term 'stress'. All kinds of sufferings are a kind of conditioned experience which arises out of clinging to desires. According to Buddhist philosophy, a compassionate person following an eightfold path can feel relieved from all the sufferings of life.

Mindfulness of breath is a powerful technique to overcome suffering. In the practice of Buddhism, we can see that all mental formations such as compassion, love, fear, sorrow, and despair are organic in nature. People can transform them through mindful breathing. There is no path to the cessation of suffering without suffering itself. Buddhism suggests to embrace our suffering and to look at it deeply in order to understand its nature. Looking at suffering deeply, we will have deep insight into its nature, and the path of transformation and healing will present itself to us.

Critical Analysis

The present chapter is an attempt to critically examine the dimensions of an individualistic society generating stress, uncertainty, and feelings of failure in the masses, which in turn generate the need for new choices in the advice and counselling industries. In order to divert the root of the problem, the experts of treatment conveniently divert the attention to individuals' responsibility for their failures.

The causes of stress among individuals should encompass a broad spectrum of factors rather than being understood with individual pathologization perspective. It may seem counter intuitive to the dominant literature and with its excessive emphasis on individuals as the responsible factors for stress but the deleterious effects of interrelated factors of economy, spirituality, ideology, technology, social inequality and contextual factors role is an undeniable reality.

Socio-cultural, technological, and economic conditions play a demonstrable role between the societal conditions and human stress, contrary to the majority of researchers focusing on individual aspects. The aspects of stark inequalities which haunt the everyday life of the billion are posing pathological conditions of obsessional neurosis. The life of a common man is full of challenges in terms of satisfying the basic needs, and majority of the middle class confronted with difficulties experience greater feelings of anxiety, inadequacy, and guilt for not being able to fulfil their fundamental expectations. Most of the people not realizing their true potential in various activities and professions regard themselves as exceptions to the rule, but, in fact, similar situations persist for many. One of the paradoxical aspects of Indian culture is the volarization of 'celebrity status' and restraint that accompanies its processes, which turns out to be a source of self-doubt because of nagging feelings of failure. Another ironical feature that perplexes the minds of a common man in India involves the ideals of spirituality, which are considered highest ideals of the life, but social realities promote achieving economically motivated objectives. The culture of choice is glorified in contemporary societies, but inherent disadvantages of education, economic status, and proximity to power create categories of disadvantage, and it becomes difficult to bridge the gaps of inequality.

The adaptation of the poor to the ladders of success is practically impossible because of poor education, poverty, and poor health, and they are outcast as others in the form of stigmatized individuals or groups.

It is an unfortunate reality in the Indian context that majority of the children do not get access to quality education and quality-health facilities, and the social condition engenders their potentials to the norms of adaptation to be successful in life barring few exceptions. Poor housing conditions, constant debt, and unemployment are important indicators which put such individuals under pressures to escape the reality of competition to be participants in the serious activities despite having potential to do so. It is not surprising to highlight that conditions of chronic poverty creates a vicious cycle inhibiting the growth of one's potential. Plight of contemporary Indian society is flecked with undesirable social conditions which many people wish to correct. American sociologist Wright Mills uses the term 'sociological imagination' to return to this ability to see the impact of social forces on individuals, especially on their private lives. Sociological study is not the same as our 'common sense', and it suggests moving from thinking about the individual and his problems and focusing on social, economic, and historical circumstances that produce the problem.

In order to understand the problems of stress, it is suggested to account for its multi-pronged origin which has structural and functional dimensions. For example the problem of homelessness does not arise out of mysterious circumstances or unemployment for which long-term structural features such as housing for all and employment for all are solutions. Social policy, advocacy, and innovation can foster changes at community level which may contribute to the wellness at individual level as well.

Summary

This chapter presents a detailed description of the term 'stress' from historical to contemporary time period. The conditions of stress can be understood from various perspectives which comprises appraisal aspects, neurological aspects, cognitive aspects, techno-stress, cultural stress, and socially embedded stress. It further explains the concepts of extended mind and the role of roles in stress causation and its precipitation. Role strain theory provides a comprehensive understanding of the gaps between individual goals and their lack of abilities to achieve those goals. In the subsequent pages, a unique differentiation of surviving poor, passive poor, retreating poor, and resisting poor presents an unique distinction category which people respond to when faced with stress. Pearlin's concept of role strain experienced by individuals' participation in social roles highlights the nature of tasks, transpersonal conflict, role captivity, adaptation, role restructuring, and interpersonal conflict.

The stress mastery is a paradoxical phenomenon which suggests that gaining mastery is a confidence booster, but in order to maintain this sense of mastery, beyond a point, people can experience stress. Lack of social diversity in a society also leads to the dominance of particular groups: groups of race, gender, religion, or any other demographic diversity factor. Social categorization has its influence on thoughts, feelings, and behaviours towards other groups. The problems of social categorization lead to distortions in our perceptions against the members of outgroups. Many false perceptions and stereotype are perpetuated in the society, which harm the self-esteem and dignity of out-groups members. Research has found that stereotype threat is caused by both cognitive and affective factors.

The concept of melting pot theory has been used to describe societies that are formed by an assortment of immigrant cultures which eventually produce new hybrid social and cultural forms. It is a monocultural metaphor for a heterogeneous society, which blends together as one Multiculturalism is an idea in which various cultural/ethnic groups interact with each other without sacrificing their unique identities. Multiculturalism is also described as salad bowl and as a cultural mosaic in which cultural pluralities co-exist with each other. The tendency to incorporate and appreciate the values of diverse culture promotes the tendency of 'live and let live' principle. In the contemporary society, so many conflicts and controversies are centred around issues of linguistic, cultural, and traditions differences, and ethnic minority group members experience stress due to these tensions. So many political parties use identity politics to in order to expand their support base which may be counterproductive to the minority group members. Technology-related developments created so many facilities for the human beings, but modern technology also became a source of stress. People are more connected than ever due to rapid advancements in technology, but overuse of technology may have adverse psychological effects including isolation, depression, and anxiety.

Every individual is inevitably immersed in a technological environment in their day-to-day activities for the fulfilment of needs relating to profession, business, and other responsibilities which may contribute to stress directly or indirectly.

Some of the stressors are structural in nature, while others exist at the level of individuals. Technological development also gives rise to alienation due to differences in power to connect with those technologies. Capitalists use technology to suit their own interests which is in the hands of corporate community with profit maximization objectives. Technology-related alienation and work stress are very common phenomena in mechanized factories. There are several instances of problems of visual and postural fatigue, headache, depressions, and sleep problems for the people working in high-tech environments. Night-shift works in media and information technology industry adversely affect the sleep cycle, resulting in health problems.

Techno stress is caused due to factors of work overload and other complexities associated with technology-related works. Digital stress is generated by the effects of Internet-mediated communication. Internet-related communication platforms have emerged as a potential source of stress for its users, which have significant indirect effects of depression, anxiety, and burnout. Excessive use of digital media network and its communication can serve as a channel for the contagion of emotion. Digital media usage is also associated with constructs like narcissism, excessive interest in self, and lower levels of empathy. The 24% of availability of digital media through persistent beeping, vibrating, and flashing of notifications keep the users engaged, and it has implications for cognitive skills, sleep disturbances, or fear of missing out on something, which gives rise to a type of social anxiety that arises from the fear that one is missing out on something. Social media by its nature promotes social comparison, and it also creates a gap between real-life activities and what is presented on social media.

In order to cope with the negative aspects, people should try to find out time to disengage from social media and set some boundaries for its absence replacing with certain meaningful family and society interactions. The unseen violence generated by capitalism is known as structural violence. It is a broad social system inherently flawed and not optimally designed to meaningfully or efficiently distribute justice, safety, or resources despite having the capability to do so (Galtung, 1969). James Gilligan defines structural violence as the increased rates of death and disability suffered by those have occupy the bottom rungs of society. It is important to understand that structural factors of deprivation contribute to the large segment of population to suffer which are preventable conditions. The pressure of being poor and consumption of food with low nutritional value are associated with negative health outcomes and mental health ailments and increased levels of stress. Poverty is a fundamental pre-condition of many negative outcomes including child abuse and depression and diarrhoea.

It would be apt to suggest that understanding the problem of stress requires multi-perspectives to be taken into account, and a mere focus on individuals as the center will not serve the purpose. A detailed and comprehensive introspection of the technological, cultural, digital, ideological modernity aspects; capitalistic analysis; and social factors analysis can help us to decode the problem and its solutions. This can be hoped that researchers involved in this area will attach more importance to the holistic understanding of this issue and come out with more realistic reflections to foresee a happier society in the real sense of the term.

Key Points:

- Stress as a result of cognitive processes focuses on appraisal systems.
- Dialogical self is a dynamic multiplicity of 'I' positions intertwined with the minds of the other people.
- Coping is considered to be a normative process.
- Role strain occurs when people are faced with gaps between their goals and current status.
- Role captivity occurs when a person experiences a discrepancy between his/her current goal and a desired goal.
- Multiculturalism is the name ascribed to belief or ideas that promote recognition, appreciation, celebration, and preservation of social differences.

- Technostress is the inability to cope with new technology in a healthy manner.
- Excessive usage of social media is a significant contributor to stress in the digital era.
- Ideology of capitalism and consumerism also results in stress.
- Melting pot theory is used to describe societies that are formed by an assortment of immigrant cultures which eventually produce new hybrid social and cultural forms.
- Engagement coping is mainly problem-focused coping.

Key Terms:

Distributed cognition, Technostress, Ergonomics, Think-act-trilogy, Jouissance, Accommodative coping, Extraversion, Resilience, Cognitive-restructuring, Mindfulness

References

Aneshensel, C. S. (2010). Neighbourhood as a social context of the stress process. In W. R. Avison et al. (Eds.), *Advances in the conceptualization of the stress process* (pp. 35–52). Springer.

Bandura A (1986). *Social foundations of thought and actions: A social cognitive theory*. Prentice-Hall.

Bord, C. C. (1984). *Technostress: The human cost of the computer revolution*. Addison-Wesley Publishing, Company.

Bossler, A. M., & Holt, T. J. (2009). Online activities, guardianship, and malware infection: An examination of routine activities theory. *International Journal of Cyber Criminology*, *3*(1), 400–420.

Bossler, A. M., Holt, T. J., & May, D. C. (2012). Predicting online harassment victimization among a juvenile population. *Youth Society*, *44*(4), 500–523.

Boyd, D. (2014). *It's complicated: The social lives of networked teens*. Yale University Press.

Brezo, J., Paris, J., & Turecki, G. (2006). Personality traits as correlates of suicidal ideation, suicide attempts, and suicide completions: A systematic review. *Acta psychiatrica scandinavica*, *113*(3), 180–206.

Campas, B. E., Cannor, J., Osoweicki, D., & Welch, A. (1997). Effortful and involuntary responses to stress: Implications for coping with chronic stress. In B. H. Gottlieb (Ed.), *Coping with chronic stress* (pp. 105–130). Plenum.

Carr, C. T., & Shayes, R. A. (2015). Social media: Defining, developing and divining. *Atlantic Journal of Communication, 23*(1), 46–65.

Carver, C. S., & Harmon-Jones, E. (2009). Anger is an approach-related affect: Evidence and implications. *Psychological Bulletin*, *135*, 183–204.

Carver, C. S., & Scheier, M. F. (1998). *On the self-regulation of behavior*. Cambridge University Press.

Carver, C. S., & Scheier, M. F. (2008). *Perspectives on personality* (6th ed.). Allyn & Balon.

Carver, C. S., Scheier, M. F., & Weintraub, J. K. (1989). Assessing coping strategies: A theoretically based approach. *Journal of Personality and Social Psychology, 56*, 267–283.

Cingel, D. P., & Krcmar, M. (2014). The amazing teen brain: What every child advocates needs to know. *Child Law Practice Newsletter, 28*(2), 21–24.

Clark, A., & Chalmers, D. (1998). The extended mind. *Analysis, 58*(1), 7–19.

Cole, P. M., Martin, S. E., & Dennis, T. A. (2004). Emotion regulation as a scientific construct: Methodological challenges and directions for child development research. *Child Development, 75*, 317–333.

Collier, A. (2014). Perspectives on parenting in a digital age. In A. B. Jordan & D. Ramer (Eds.), *Media and well-being of children and adolescent*s (pp. 247–264). Oxford University Press.

Compas, B. E., Cannor, J. K., Saltzman, H., Thomson, A. H., & Wadsworth, M. (1999). Getting specific about coping: Effortful and involuntary responses to stress in development. In M. Lewis & D. Ramsay (Eds.), *Soothing and stress* (pp. 229–256). Erlbaum.

Compass, B. E., Cannor-Smith, J. K., Saltzman, H., Thomson, A. H., & Wadsworth, M. E. (2001). Coping with stress during childhood and adolescence: Problem, progress and potential in theory and research. *Psychological Bulletin, 127*, 87–127.

Connor-Smith, J. K., & Flachsbart, C. (2007). Relations between personality and coping: A meta-analysis. *Journal of Personality and Social Psychology, 93*(6), 1080.

Cooper, C. L., & Dew, P. (2004). *Stress: A brief history*. Blackwell Publishing Ltd.

Deci, E. L., & Ryan, R. M (1985). *Intrinsic motivation and self-determination in human behavior*. Plenum.

Eder, M. D. (1916). An address on the psychopathology of war neuroses. *Lancet, 191*, 264–268.

Elliot, A. J. (Ed.). (2008). *Handbook of approach and avoidance motivation*. Psychology Press.

Federici, S. (2013). With philosophy and terror: Transforming bodies into labor power. In A. Marvakis et al. (Eds.), *Doing psychology under new conditions concord* (pp. 2–10). Captus Press Inc.

Focault, M. (1980). *The history of sexuality, volume 1: An introduction*. Vintage Books.

Forsyth, D. (1915). Functional nerve disease and the shack of battle: A study of so called traumatic neuroses arising in Connection of the war. *Lancet, 189*, 1399–1403.

Galtung, J. (1969). Violence, peace and peace research. *Journal of Peace Research* Vol 6, No. 3.

Green, C. S., & Bavelier, D. (2003). Action video game modifies visual selective attention. *Nature, 423*, 534–537.

Grinker, R. R., & Spiegel, J. P. (1945). *Men under stress* (2nd ed.). Blakiston. ASIN B000061Z5Y.

Hermans, H. J. M. (2001). The construction of a personal position repertoire: Method and practice. *Culture & Psychology*, 7(3), 323–365.

Higgins, E. T. (1996). Ideas, ought and regulatory focus: Affect and motivation from distinct pains and pleasures. In P. M. Gollwitzer & J. A. Barg (Eds.), *The psychology of action: Linking cognition and motivation behavior* (pp. 91–114). Guilford.

Hutchins, E. (1995). *Cognition in the wild*. Bradford.

Kakar, S. (1979). The inner world: A psychoanalytic study of childhood and society in India. *The Journal of Asian Studies, 38*, 795–796.

Kessler, R. C., Angermeyer, M., Anthony, J. C. et al. (2007). Lifetime prevalence and age-of-onset distributions of mental disorders in the world health organization's world mental health survey initiative. *World Psychiatry*, *6*, 168–176.

Kim-Cohen, J. et al. (2003). Prior juvenile diagnoses in adults with mental disorder: Developmental follow-back of a prospective-longitudinal cohort. *Archives of General Psychiatry*, *60*, 709–717.

Klein, A.-M., Vaissiere, B. E., Cane, J. H., Steffan-Dewenter, I., Cunningham, S. A., Kremen, C., & Tscharntke, T. (2007). Importance of pollinators in changing landscapes for world crops. *Proceedings of the Royal Society B, Biological Sciences*, *274*(1608), 303–313.

Kopp, C. B. (1989). Regulation of distress and negative emotions: A developmental view. *Developmental Psychology*, *25*, 343–354.

Lazarus, R. S. (1966). *Psychological stress and the coping process*. McGraw Hill.

Lazarus, R. S., & Ericksen, C. W. (1952). *Effects of failure stress upon skilled*. Journal of Experimental Psychology. 43: 100-5. PMID 14927807 DOI: 10.1037/H0056614.

Lazarus, R. S., & Folkman, S. (1984). *Stress appraisal and coping*. Springer Pub. Co.

Leader, D. (2008). *The new black: Mourning Melancholia and depression*. Hamish Hamilton.

Linell, P. (2009). *Rethinking language, mind and world dialogically: International and Contextual theories of human sense making: A volume in cultural psychology: Constructing human development*. Information Age.

Markova, T. (2006). On the inner alter in dialogue. *International Journal for Dialogical Science*, *1*(1), 125–147.

Mechanic, D. (1974). Social Structure and personal adaptation: Some neglected dimensions. In G. V. Cohello, D. Hamburg, & J. E. Adams (Eds.), *Coping and adaptation* (pp. 32–44). Basic Books.

Meier, B. P., & Robinson, M. D. (2004). Does quick to blame mean quick to anger? The role of agreeableness in dissociating blame and anger. *Personality and Social Psychology Bulletin*, 856–867.

Merton, R. (1938). Social structure and Anomie. *American Sociological Review*, *3*(5), 672–682.

Metcalfe, J., & Mischel, W. (1999). A hot/cool-system analysis of delay of gratification: Dynamics of will power. *Psychological Review*, *106*, 3–19.

Moos, R. H., & Schaefer, J. A. (1993). Coping resources and processes: Current concept and measures. In L. Goldberger & S. Brenitz (Eds.), *Handbook of stress: Theoretical and clinical aspects* (pp. 234–257). Free Press.

Parker, H. N. (2011). Toward a definition of popular culture. *History and Theory*, *50*, 147–170.

Pearlin, L. I. (1983). Role strains and personal stress. In H. B. Kaplan (Ed.), *Psychological stress; Trends in theory and research* (pp. 3–32). Academic.

Pearlin, L. I. (1991). The study of coping: Problems and directions. In J. Eckenrode (Ed.), *The social context of coping* (pp. 261–276). Plenum Press.

Pearlin, L. I., & Bierman (2013). Current issues and future directions in research into the stress process. In *Handbook of the sociology of mental health* (2nd ed., pp. 325–340). Springer.

Roth, S., & Cohen, L. J. (1986). Approach, avoidance, and coping with stress. *American Psychologist*, *41*(7), 813–819.

Rothbart, M. K., Derryberry, D., & Posner, M. I. (1994). A psychobiological approach to the development of temperament. In J. E. Bates & T. D. Wachs

(Eds.), *Temperament: Individual difference at the interface of biology and behavior* (pp. 83–116). American Psychological Association.
Salecl, R. (2010). *The tyranny of choice*. Profile Books Ltd.
Skinner, E. A., Edge, K., Altman, J., & Sherwood, H. (2003). Searching for the structure of coping: A review and critique of category system for classifying ways of coping. *Psychological Bulletin, 129*, 216–269.
Steel, P., Schmidt, J., & Shultz, J. (2008). Refining the relationship between personality and subjective well-being. *Psychological Bulletin, 134*, 138–161.
Turkle, S. (2015). *Reclaiming conversation: The power of talk in a digital age*. Penguin Books
Valkenburg, P. M., Schouten, A. P., & Peter, J. (2005). Adolescents' identity experiments on the internet. *New Media and Society*, 7, 383–402.
Valsiner, J. (2007). *Culture in minds and societies. Foundation of cultural psychology*. Sage Publication.
Valsiner, J. (1998). *The guided mind*. Harvard University Press.
Viner, R. (1999). Putting stress in life: Hans Selye and the making of stress theory. *Social Studies of Science, 29*(3), 391–410.
Weinstein, E. C., Selman, R. L., Thomas, S., Kim, J.-E., White, A. E., & Dinakar, K. (2016). How to cope with digital stress: The recommendations adolescents offer their peers online. *Journal of Adolescents Research, 31*(4), 415–441.
WHO (2017, May). *Diarrhoeal disease*. WHO.

3 Ecology and Well-being

Learning Objectives

After reading this chapter, you will be able to understand:

- Ecology and well-being
- Ecological well-being and mental health
- Eco-system approach
- Indian approach to ecology and well-being

Introduction

What Is ecology? What Is Its Relevance in the Present Time?

Psychological well-being (PWB) is a superordinate construct that includes emotional or psychological well-being as well as social and collective well-being. The term 'quality of life' is similar to psycho-social well-being in that it involves emotional, social, and physical components.

Measures of well-being are sometimes divided into objective measures, which mostly refer to 'standard of living', and subjective measures incorporate psychological, social, ecological, and spiritual judgements individuals make about their lives. It is a multidimensional construct which is much broader and includes other aspects related to mental and physical health like perceived stress. Psychological well-being is a central concept and relevant in the areas of research related to epidemiology and its implications for health outcomes.

The main dimensions of PWB include hedonic well-being (feeling happy); evaluative well-being (being satisfied with life); eudaimonic well-being (e.g. finding purpose is life, having a sense of mastery and autonomy in one's decisions); and constructs of optimism, hope, resilience, and self-efficacy.

PWB dimensions are potential contributors to illness and wellness aspects of individuals. The factors of personal growth, mastery, purpose in life, autonomy, life satisfaction, sense of coherence, and other dimensions of PWB spectrum such as socio-economic status and ecological well-being

DOI: 10.4324/9781003350651-3

too have been studied in relationship to health dimensions, and it has been found to impact the decline in levels of stress cardiometabolic diseases and reduce overall mortality of individuals.

It has also been found that only a small proportion of PWB factors are explained by dispositional/heritable factors, and a large proportion of environmental or ecological influences can account for a large part of an individual's well-being.

There have been various well-being surveys conducted based on relevant indices of environment and landscape factors, social relationship's probing meaningful activities and relationships with positive/negative affect. Such surveys also issue annual 'happiest country on earth' list, recognizing certain well-being measures as a reliable indicator of overall citizen satisfaction.

The term 'ecology' coming from a Greek word meaning 'household' is the branch of biology that studies relationship between organisms and their surroundings with regard to the adaptations of organisms to the environments and the resulting population distributions. Ecology also aims to study the invasion and succession among communities and the replacement of one species by another that are more suitable to the changed environment.

The term 'psychological ecology' was introduced by Lewis with an emphasis on environment factors more than the individual factor to understand organisms–environment relationships. Lewis came up with his famous approach to explain human behaviour as a function of the person and environment and the concept of life-space (Lewin, 1942–44, p. 169). Based on Gestalt principles of field theory, the constituents of life space are the forces that are against each other leading to conflict situations and life barriers, which also impinge on behaviour.

Lewin (1931) distinguished between the scientific concepts of Aristotle and Galileo and argued that Galilean science stresses the relation of an object with its environment whereas Aristotelian science classifies objects on the basis of inner essence.

This shift from Aristotelian to Galilean science had taken place in physics and biology, and its implications in psychology and human behaviour were highlighted by Lewin with reference to Einstein; Lewin defined a field as 'a totality of coexisting facts which are conceived of as mutually interdependent' (Lewin, 1946, p. 729). Every region in the field holds positive or negative valences, showing their attractive or repulsive character. Lewin also talked about conflict situations and barriers and the concept of driving forces towards a positive or negative. In a plus-plus conflict, a person is located between two positive valences, and, in a minus-minus conflict, a person is located between two negative valences (Lewin, 1946)

In a plus-minus conflict situation, incompatible forces from the same region act upon a person, exemplified as the 'promise of reward for doing a disagreeable task' (Lewin, 1946, p. 809f).

Person–environment analysis provides a useful contribution to understand the impact of contextual and environmental factors as facilitating or impeding factors in well-being. This approach is useful in analysing how person environment can influence the working conditions and well-being of people at work.

It is widely recognized that natural and biodiversity impacts have important repercussions for human health and well-being. For example disturbance of ecosystem and in particular biodiversity loss may affect human health through an increase in the spread of zoonotic diseases (Keesing et al., 2010; Ostfeld & Keesing, 2000) or through losses of pharmacological opportunity (Chivian et al., 2008).

Cultural ecosystems services have been defined as the 'non-material' benefits that are derived from ecosystem and are related to factors such as promotion of well-being through aesthetics, leisure and recreation and sense of place (Churich et al., 2011).

Environmental degradation, including biodiversity loss, appears to exert adverse impacts on health, especially mental well-being, which is more dangerous than the adverse effects caused due to economic decline, nutritional deficiency, and pollution (Speldewinde et al., 2009).

Health and environmental awareness organizations suggest the significance of roles of clean air, clean water, and natural ecosystem in the promotion of good health and psychological well-being. Theoretical underpinnings and conceptual frameworks consistently suggest environment–health linkages with researchers in different disciplines. In the field of social science studies, the biophilia hypothesis (Kellert & Wilson, 1995), attention restoration, and psycho-evolutionary stress theories (Ulrich et al., 1991) describe the potentially innate connection of humans with the natural world, indicating that greater exposure leads to better health outcomes. Several other factors like the impact of neighbourhood, increased level of vegetation, and role of architecture are also positively associated with the measures of well-being.

The biodiversity changes caused due to pollution, habitat destruction, and climate change result in adverse effects on health and well-being.

Gibson's Ecological Psychology

The term ecological psychology is strongly associated with James and Eleanor J. Gibson's approach to study perception and Roger Barker's approach to study social interactions. The origin of both these approaches lies in the contribution of James who highlighted the importance of everyday experience. **Ecopsychology** studies the relationship between the well-being of individuals and that of the planet.

Gibson (2002) emphasized two concept of affordances, which he considered as opportunities for action created by match between environmental properties and organism properties. Gibson argued that perception is highly influenced by environmental surroundings. Perception is an active process, and it is more accurate when people are allowed to move more freely. Affordances are meant to describe that in different situations, different actions are possible.

Thus, individuals are able to perceive the affordances in terms of relative evolutionary and developmental factors. From the perspective of affordance concept, one can identify the properties of the organisms and the environment that determine which actions are possible. According to Gibson's tradition, organisms successfully match their behaviour with the environment because they learn to discriminate between complex patterns of energy that specify which actions are possible. Gibson (1979) argued from this approach that perceptual explanations of individuals can be used to solve cognitive tasks. However, Gibson's theoretical explanations could not explain more sophisticated solutions to classic perceptual problems.

Barker's Ecological Psychology

Objective reality theory puts emphasis on objective reality aspects of the environment with observalite geographical, physical, and temporal attributes.

Barker's conception of ecological psychology can be described on the basis of important assumptions: 1) the system of relationship that links individuals and groups with their social and physical environment is complex; ii) such systems can't be understood in isolated functions; iii) environment–behaviour systems develop and change over long periods of times; and iv) the challenges of ecological psychology require an understanding of environmental systems to predict the interventions (Barker & Grump, 1964).

Behavioural settings that are common to a person's day-to-day life experiences produce no difficulties in recognizing and linking ecological psychology to readily understood concepts. Human and physical component interaction in a synchronized fashion is known as behavioural setting.

Barker's concept of ecological psychology has been applied in practical situations.

The natural units of environment are called behavioural settings discovered through observation. Large-scale inventories of behavioural settings can reveal changes in the quality of life of a community, and surveys for behavioural settings can be conducted in a variety of locations such as schools, workplaces, religious places, or retail shops. Some theories use an ecological perspective to study urban crime. While Barker had emphasized commodities among behavioural settings of the same type, other theorists have focused on the uniqueness of the settings.

Environmental psychologist Barker emphasized on leaving laboratory and having more reliance on naturalistic observation. The effects of context or situation upon behaviour have been recognized in the works of Milgram's and Zimbardo's simulated prison research.

Ecological principles for embedded behaviour

Traditional cognitive science approach focus is that behaviour is an outcome of representation-based information processing systems. Organisms and environment make an inseparable pair, which is a key element in the behavioural outcome. Just as the twentieth-century biologists described and measured the environment at home for life, ecological psychologists described the environment of home for perceiving and acting. It is worthwhile to appreciate ecologists niches, dens, predators which constitute a fundamental ontology. Real (objective, measurable) that constitutes the environment and its measurements of environment (e.g. Hordances) and together it shapes the property of the environment. Ecological psychology perspective of information means a pattern in space and time that specifies a state of affairs of the organism–environment system. The concept of perception an action in ecological psychology.

The behaviour of an individual cannot be independent of the geographical environment. The manifestations of behavioural environment rest on the existence of certain properties of the geographical environment. 'Life is a series of locations as the body traces it paths through space' (Mc Ginn, 1999, p. 106). Psychology is considered handicapped owing to its emphasis on physicalism which treats qualities of human experience as epiphenomenal, and subjectivists consider the environment as so many individually experienced cognitive constructions.

Behaviour settings is a broad term indicating a number of environmental features that have varying degrees of influence on behaviour. Following R. Barker (1968, pp. 16–17), behaviour settings include characteristics as stated in the following paragraph. Behaviour setting, like Gibson's terms 'perceptual systems' and 'affordance', is often used in the literature in imprecise ways.

Behaviour setting have a specifiable geographical location and temporal boundaries that are self-generated and maintained by the dynamics of their occupants. The boundaries of behaviour settings are discriminate – that is they can be perceived.

Behavioural settings are quasi-stable as they manifest mechanisms in response to perturbations, and in so doing, they preserve their integrity within limits.

Behavioural settings exist independently of any single person's experience of them. Individuals who occupy a particular behaviour setting are interdependent by an appreciable degree.

According to Barker's terminology, behaviour settings are 'circumfacent' to (their surrounding) individual behaviour. The meaning of a behaviour setting is determined by the kind of activities happening in a place. Behaviour settings as places afford certain possibilities for an individual. Individuals selectively engage particular kind of affordances in their surroundings and selectively seek out certain behaviour settings. The synomorphy of milieu and behaviour rises due to an explicit demand of behaviour for a particular milieu. The term synomorphy refers to the presence of congruence between topographic features of the setting and behavioural activities taking place in the setting. The meaning of behavioural settings is situated in perceived synomorphic relations between milieu features and action.

Ecological Knowledge

Meaningful features of common environments grant out of social processes and socio-historical contexts. Environment comprises meaningful objects, meaningful places, and institutions, and these features of shared environment have been collectively created by us. Ecological knowledge suggests many individual and collective discoveries, and they take place in a dynamic, cumulative process. Many things that we know and wish to know are woven into the public sphere of our socio-cultural world. It is important to understand the public nature of ecological knowledge, which empowers our potential as social individuals.

The Ecology of Culture

Cultural systems are an ongoing process in which an individual is born. Individuals enter into a world whose meanings are relatively determined through collective actions, and they also try to contribute for its transformation.

The concept of structuration suggests that the notion of collective social processes produces social structures. There is a 'duality of structures' (Shotter) in the sense that the structural properties of social systems are both medium and outcome of the practice they recursively organize (P. 25). Bourdieu (1977) conceptualized individual psychological functioning as a system of dispositions to act (habitus), which has been brought into existence by structures constituting the individual's 'material conditions of existence' (P. 72). It is suggested by prominent theories that individuals find themselves in a world that has been constructed by their predecessors and that they in turn tend to sustain.

In the relation between biological and socio-cultural processes that later factors play a more constitutive and humanizing role in an individual's development. Humans independent of culture can exhibit unchanneled monstrosities with lesser instincts and lack of sentiments. Undirected by cultural patterns, a man's behaviour would be virtually ungovernable, a mere chaos of pointless acts and exploding emotions, and his experience shapeless. Culture, accumulated totality of such patterns, is not just an ornament of human existence but the principal basis of its specificity – an essential condition of it (Geertz, 1973, p. 46). Evidence from archaeological sources indicate that the evolution of modern human was strongly influenced by the cultural processes.

Urban Ecology and Well-being

What is a city? A simple working definitions is:

On inhabited central place differentiated from a town or village by its greater size and by the range of activities practiced within its boundaries usually religious, military, political, economic, educational and cultural. Collectively, these activities involves the exercise of power over the surrounding. Country side (Jary & Jary, 1999) Urban centres are spaces where a large number of people live in close proximity in which the majority of the contacts are fleeting and partial.

There are certain characteristics of urban life such as pace of life and competition, which tend to prevail over cooperation. The urban way of life weaken the bonds of kinship, and make the tradition of families and communities less prominent. Cities are mostly artificial environments constructed by people. The process of industrialization contributed to the growth of urbanization and the movement of people away from indigenous areas. The migration in India resulted due to unemployment in the villages and poor people moving to cities in search of secured jobs.

The rapidly expanding cities and megacities are faced with environmental problems of pollution, housing shortages, inadequate sanitation, unsafe water, and chronic health problems.

Migrants labourers in India crowd into squatter zones, which mushroom around the edge of cities. Some of the largest slum dwelling areas in Dharavi, Mumbai, or Jahangirpuri in Delhi are inhabited by millions of migrant labourers, what has been called the 'septic fringe' of the urban areas. Congestion on the roads, vehicular pollution and industrial pollution leads to serious health hazards.

A direct link between the amount of accessible local green space and health has also been evidenced using large-scale epidemiological studies.

Walking in parks and engaging in exercises can positively contribute towards better health outcomes.

Access to green spaces is considered to promote healthy living through participation in activities like walking, jogging, and cycling.

Levels of aggression and violence were also significantly higher for residents staying in conditions lacking vegetations than for those who had access to nature (Kuo & Sullivan, 2001). Access to greener pastures reduces aggression through the impact of mediating factors such as exercise, walking, and recreational activities at such places. Therefore, neighbourhood settings lacking access to nature and greenery had a significant effect on human social functioning.

Environmental architecture and aesthetics are positively associated with well-being. The levels of engagement with nature in terms of viewing and functional and active participation can lead to different levels of satisfaction among its users. Windows present in the work place can buffer the stresses of work and reduce the frequency of illness, headaches, and frustration and improve patience and enthusiasm for work (Leather et al., 1998; Kaplan, 2001). Workers allowed to wear casual dresses and working in workplaces decorated with flowers have been shown to feel less stressed in their jobs and to derive greater job satisfaction than workers overlooking built environments. Two classic and widely cited studies from 1980s (Moore, 1982; Ulrich, 1984) suggest that prolonged exposure to window views of nature can have important health-related consequences.

The first study found that prisoners in Michigan, USA, whose cells overlooked farmland and forests, reported 24% lesser sick cell visits as compared with those in cells facing prison yard. The second 'classical' study configuration of a hospital in Pennsylvania was analysed in which surgical rooms were facing deciduous trees and other set of rooms were facing brick wall. In the record of surgery patients of last 10 years with identical surgeries, hospital stay was shorter for the patients with tree views as compared to the patients staying in rooms facing brick wall.

This can be reasonably assumed on the basis of large numbers of empirical studies available in this area that environmental factors significantly contribute to the attention perception, concentration, and emotional restoration aspects of human health and well-being. Mental health and overall well-being get seriously affected with the crowding.

In urban areas, less access to nature and green space is a significant contributor to human health and well-being.

The Ecosystem Approach

Ecosystems approach is an integrated management strategy of land, water, and living resources aimed at promoting conservation and sustainable utilization of genetic resources. Eco-system approach further means a dynamic complex plan of living organisms and non-living environment interacting as a functional unit.

Ecosystem approach does not rely on rigid conservation approaches and contain elements of learning by doing depending upon the contextual situations.

Social, biological, and cultural diversity presents a diverse character of ecosystem approach being viewed differently from a stakeholder's point of view. The rationale for ecosystem approach focuses upon equal participation *by* its stakeholders including indigenous and local communities in the decision-making process. Balancing the interest of multiple communities requires transparent and nested nature of decisions at the grassroots level.

The ecosystem approach to health is a promising strategy which considers that human health and well-being are results of dynamic interactions of people with social, cultural economic, and natural environment.

Assuming health to be a complex outcome of interdependent factors of social, cultural, and environmental well-being, the relationship between man and nature acquires a crucial importance.

Health and well-being of people are strongly influenced and affected by geographical factors and a variety of biological, social, and psychological factors emerging in a particular context.

Socio-environmental conflicts are increasingly visible in society, and the complexity of their solutions has posed new challenges to the scientists, researchers, and practitioners of this field.

There are numerous examples of harmful effects in human health caused by pollutants such as dioxins and pesticides. In the ecosystem approach, various sectors of economy, ecology, community, and environments are integrated for achieving better outcomes. This approach provides opportunities for appreciation of learning by differing knowledge bases.

Trans-disciplinarity is a key characteristic of the ecosystem approach, which involves multiple stakeholders leading to the development of novel dimensions to resolve environment mental problems.

Another important pillar of ecosystem approach is the adoption of eco-health-equity in which the interest of all sectors, regardless of gender or socio-economic status, is taken into account.

Ecosystem approach as a strategy has become a very effective method striving to achieve the mission and sustainable use of ecosystem.

The United Nations Environment Programme (UNEP) has called for widespread introduction of marine spatial planning (MSP) indicating growing concern about the state of our seas which is resulting in development of new approaches to marine planning and management.

Indian Approach: Indian Perspective of Environment

The reverence to nature and its unifying ethical principles occupy a great importance in traditional Indian culture. All social and cultural activities in the ancient Indian society suggest a complete harmony of human beings with five elements of nature. The earth, water, air, light, and cosmos have been worshipped as Gods in reality and symbolically, a tradition which exists till date. People in India worship peepal trees (*Ficus religiosa*) and coconut trees (*Cocus nucifera*) with a belief that women who nurse the desire to get a son worship coconut trees and eat coconut fruits as a 'divine gift'.

The primitive societies of India represented by the tribals (aborigines) living in mountains and forests have significantly contributed towards the protection of several virgin forests rich in biodiversity called 'sacred groves' (Forest God) and are left untouched by the local people.

The intrusion in such reserved forests, usually dedicated to a deity, is considered as a taboo, and intruders may be punished with its violation. Many sacred graves are found in Himalayan region, and one such region found near in Chakrata (Dehradun) is known as Deoban (Forest of Gods).

Vedas

The harmony between *jal*, *vayu*, and *agni* (water, air, and fire) is considered to be like as members of a family, and any kind of damage done to anyone can result in the destruction of the human beings according to the tenets of Rigvedic philosophy. Rivers flowing in their natural stream should neither be polluted nor the trees on its banks should be cut off or uprooted. Ancient treasure of Vedic knowledge has several traditions related to protection of *paryavaran* (environment) lying between dyaus (heavens) and *prithvi* (earth).

The Rigveda venerates deities like *Mitra* and *Varuna*. *Indra*, *Maruts*, and *Aditya* are considered to be responsible for maintaining the balance of nature.

Vedas speak of the integral unity of creation and the inter-connectedness or co-dependence of everything to everything else. The importance of sun is highlighted in its majestic presence in the heavens.

The sun is described in Rigveda as 'The cosmic eye, the auspicious surya mounts, upward for the good of all. The God, the eye of varuna and Mitra, Has rolled up darkness like a hide' (Rigveda VH, 62:1: deNicolas, 1976, p. 213).

This universe is not considered as a creation of random chaos, but it is considered to have a tremendous inner order and unity with an inexorable law and purpose (Rta) that govern the working of both the macrocosm and microcosm (Dandekar, 1979, p. 15). Rta is accorded highest importance in Vedic tradition determining the place, entitlement, function, and the end of everything.

Rta is also considered to be harmonious and ordered truth of being or reality which can only be discerned by the cosmic person (*purusha*).

In the tenth mandala of the Rigveda, Agni is accorded higher praise for its role in energizing subtle life forms by forming the necessary bridge between father-sky (*dyauh pitu*) and mother-earth (*prithvi mutd*).

According to Rigveda, the holy pair (Heavens and Earth) of great power moved by Rta has copulated giving birth to a child in the form of *Agni*.

Gita: By the rule of Karma, one of the central features of traditional Indian thinking does not differentiate or discriminate between humans and non-human life forms. A famous basic tenet of Indian tradition 'as one sows so one reaps' is frequently used in social interactions in day-to-day life. self, realization in Gita counters the principle of *Lokasamgraha* (the well-being of all) as a cardinal feature of its teachings.

Sankara commented, he who sees that what is painful and pleasant to himself is painful and pleasant to all creatures will cause no-living beings pain and that he who is non-injurious is the foremost of Yogins (Bilimoria &

Hutchins, 1988, p. 366). The concept of *swadharma* or working in agreement with the law of one's being and social order is considered to be divine. It is necessary to understand the focus of Gita teachings in the unity of man with the nature and with the spirit of the whole.

Jainism and Buddhism

The fundamental principle of Jainism is that every entity in the world possesses *Jiva* or sentient principle, and there are countless number of *Jivas*, which are characterized by their feature of consciousness. Scholars strongly relate the principle of *ahimsa* (non-violence) with the disciplinary ethics of Jainism. It is also argued that Jain ethic of non-injury and a compassionate regard for others support the view of interconnectedness of all *Jivas*. According to ethics of Buddhism, human beings and nature should be treated in a mode of synthesis. Buddhism codes of ethics lay a strong emphasis upon self-control, assistance, patience, contentment, purity, truthfulness, and right attitudes indicating a non-anthropocentric respect for biodiversity.

Strong application of Indian tradition of respect to plants, rivers, and animals influenced the famous approach of *sarvodaya* (welfare for all adopted by Mahatma Gandhi's environmental awareness programme). Gandhi advocated *ahimsa* (non-violence) as an instrument for social change integrating with his concept of *satyagrah* (truth) suggesting a strong preference for vegetarianism.

An important social movement towards environmental protection known as Chipko (cling onto) movement was launched by Sundar Lal Bahuguna, which involved an unrelenting action of embracing trees for preventing their felling.

Indian culture is a classic example of concept of human life in a continuity of relations between mind, body, and soul perceived in the symbiotic balance between human and natural resources. The concept of ecological balance is manifested in the feeling of divinity in all beings. The status of mother is accorded to Earth, and animals such as cows are worshiped as mothers. Blessings of cow are sought for prosperity in all endeavours and fulfilment of spiritual aspirations. The epic of *Ramayana* emphasizes on the importance of protecting the plant diversity. In the mythological story of *Ramayana,* during the war between Lord Rama and Ravana, Rama's brother, Lakshmana, falls ill and faints due to the impact of weapons, who is cured by 'Sanjeevani' herb brought by lord Hanuman.

Varaha Mihira (5th CAD) in his *Brihat Samhita* offered cues to the onset of disastrous Tsunamis as explained in chapter *Udakargaladhyaya.*

Celebrated Indian author, Kautilya, in his *Arthashashtra,* suggested suitable punishment for tree fellers and animal poachers.

The practice of 'vanmahotsava' (tree plantation ceremony) is centuries-old tradition in India. Mango and banana leaves are frequently used in majority of worshipping rituals and considered auspicious for the entry of newly wed couples used in sacred rituals of weddings. Worshipping peepal plants (*Ficus religiosa*) and banyan (*Ficus benghalensis*) on a regular basis is a very common practice in the Indian context.

It is a very remarkable feature of the Indian traditions to worship rivers. Accordingly, people gather in millions on the banks of River Ganges, which is accorded divinity status, to take a holy dip on several occasions. One such festival associated with taking holy dips in the Ganges is called Kumbh mela (Kumbh fair) which happens every 6 years as Ardh Kumbh mela and every 12 years as Kumbh mela. The cities of Prayagraj and Haridwar attract millions of devotes during the holy month of Kumbh, where people from all over the world visit to take a holy dip.

The normative value of worshipping rivers and trees is placed so high that people do not pollute or cut them, attaching a high moral duty to preserve them.

Everything related to many rivers, trees, and animals is treated as being sacred, indicating a high-level cosmic integrity of humans in Indian socio-cultural context. Varieties of rituals and elements of sacred attached with plants, herbs, rivers, and animals to restore the possible loss to ecological frameworks. However, the growth of industrialization and urbanization has resulted in the depletion of ecological framework.

Indian culture characterizes a moral duty of its citizens to protect the nature and its resources from a moral and spiritual point of view, which is extremely rare in other cultures.

Critical Evaluation

Our worsening environmental problems can be understood with a deeper understanding of ecological psychology. Burning our tropical forests releases huge amounts of carbon dioxide, which is joined by emissions from automobiles, fossil fuels, and driver technologies creating greenhouses gases. Our clean water supply is shrinking, ground water, lakes, rivers, and oceans are being polluted by the release of toxic chemicals from industrialization. The rapid growth of urbanization, desertification, and population has reduced the harvest area per person significantly in past few decades. Rain water is not in a capacity to replenish aquifers because deforestation, overgrazing, and urbanization make it more likely that water will run out. The spectre of global warming is looming large on the human civilization. An increase of the climate temperature even by a few degrees would produce devastating impact on our current habitat. Sea levels may rise owing to ecological imbalances, releasing more greenhouse gases with the danger of spreading tropical diseases. Atmospheric scientists have warned of global warming due to air pollution also eating away our ozone layer, which functions as a protective skin encircling our planet earth. Production of chlorofluorocarbons (CFCs) used in a variety of industrial production of freezers and air conditioners is likely to contribute in damaging the human immune system. In the light of several environmental issues and related damages, associated pro-environmental strategies on short-term and long-term bases are required. We must invent methods to reduce our energy consumption. The sustainable culture and common-sensical view of treating nature as a resource for our present and future need to be adopted. Psychological dimensions of our assumptions to treat human-environmental interactions in a complimentary way. We can regain our blessed place in creation by learning to co-exist with nature and not trying to control it. It is ironical that the metaphor of tree is chosen to indicate the might of expansionist powerful nations, and millions of trees are cut for human settlements and consequently denied the space for air and earth. In traditional societies, people live in groups of closely knit relationships, and the events of natural world had enormous impact on the well-being of people. In the Indian society and other traditional societies, nature is seen as a living organism, most often as mother, which is nurturing and beneficent and sometimes wild, violent, and chaotic. The image of mother earth as a living organism acts as a cultural restraint restricting the damaging human actions. One does not readily harm a mother, mutilate her body, who is considered to be alive and a sensitive topic to humans. For most traditional and spiritual societies, damage to mother earth is considered a breach of human ethical behaviour. Indian culture celebrates numerous festivals dedicated to the respect and devotion associated with the worship of plants, animals, cattle, and harvest. The Rongali Bihu coinciding with Assamese New Year reflects deep influences and connectivity with the nature. Makar Sankranti or Magh Sankranti is the day considered when there is the transition of the sun into Capricorn and is dedicated to deity Surya (Sun). Makar Sankranti is regarded an important spiritual day, and people in large numbers take dip in the holy rivers of the Ganges, Yamuna, Godavari, Krishna, and Kaveri, and it is believed that taking a holy dip on this day will result in absolution of past sins. Pongal is a multiday Hindu harvest festival dedicated to the Sun god. On the occasion of Mattu Pongal, cattle are worshipped with garlands of flowers placed on their necks. Lohri is celebrated in Punjab and Northern India, which marks the beginning of harvest season.

According to *Vedas*, *Puranas*, and other mythological texts, there is no separate existence of man apart from the duty of man to protect nature and accept what nature offers. The divine Vedic hymns provide a rich illustration of ecocentrism and strongly associate with the worship of nature. Indian concept of human–nature relationship is different from the Western perspective of anthropocentrism. The concepts of industrialism, capitalism, and consumerism pose a great risk to the symbolic relation of humans with the nature. Many of our important poets envisaged the concept of an idealistic world of man–nature relationship and deep eco-consciousness.

The problem of mental health is a result of broad spectrums of factors and their impact on human beings. The scientific understanding of ecology enriches the idea of interdependence between people and nature, which is crucial for the well-being of humans. Environmental, social, and economic resources play a crucial role to sustain emotional and physical well-being among people to satisfy their needs. Mental health and illness are dynamically associated processes with the ecology, and the extra-individual eco units serve as context for understanding the individual behaviour. Behavioural ecology orientation draws upon the coalescence of two broad perspectives – behavioural approach derived from psychology of the individual and ecological approach encompassing the study of environments.

Ecological model of mental health provides an alternative and potent approach to a person-centred causal explanation of mental health problems. This approach tends to focus on natural systems, moral behaviours, and reciprocal aspects of wellness/illness between people and their ecological contexts. Ecological perspective of well-being also focuses upon transactional aspects of person–environment fit which is dynamically related to each other. When there is a congruence or match between individuals and environments in terms of demands and their resources, a healthy outcome can be predicted. In case of an incongruence in which person–environment adaptations are misfit, it may result in unhealthy outcomes. With the active support of social intervention programmes such as controlling noise, pollution, and other relevant factors, person–environment fit can be improved.

By assuming a reciprocal impact process between people and their environments, intervention programmes can focus on modifications, facilitating a design which can promote mental health aspects. The ecosystem perspective designs the services, policies, and programmes involving the participation of local communities and people. Enhancing and enriching the values supporting the cultural diversity can lead to effective outcomes of ecology–behaviour perspective.

The ecological model also suggests that agreement on values with the affected communities can contribute to the adaptation of a harmonious approach of person–environment fit. It is a wholistic approach emphasizing linkages between persons and their environment as forming an integrated whole and a change in one part can influence changes in other parts.

The understanding of environmental domains also consists understanding social environment in addition to the intra-psychic individual factors to strengthen natural support system that influences mental health.

Albee's (1980) competence model considers human problems as resulting from an interaction between environmental stress and competence (i.e. one's ability to cope with stress) and is an alternative to 'mental defect' or 'sickness model'.

Psychological sense of community can be enhanced by strengthening factors of interdependence and shared sense of relationship with the nature, which lead to promotion of mental health. Ecologically oriented anthropologists have also considered culture as being part of a large, comprehensive network of relationships – the ecosystem. The ecological approach in anthropology is concerned with determining relationships between the natural physical environment and cultural processes (Geertz, 1966).

The economic dimensions, sociological dimensions, and ecological dimensions can collectively contribute to the mental health and well-being.

Summary

This chapter on ecology and well-being presents major synthesis of ideas, theories, research, and application, guiding the relationships between ecology and mental health.

In its first section, it provides the idea of ecology and psychological well-being. In its next section, the major theoretical conceptualizations related to ecological psychology, urban ecology, and environmental architecture and their roles in the development of maladaptive behaviour have been explained in detail.

The ecosystem approach as an integrated management strategy has been discussed highlighting the importance of indigenous and local communities' involvement in the decision-making process.

It is interesting to suggest that modern knowledge of environment popularized by Lamarck, Herbert Spencer with the translation of the milieu of Comte and Charles Darwin origin of species writing of circumstances and surroundings. But the Ancient Indian theory of environment and ecology dates back to thousands of years, constituting an integral association with nature and its various resources.

Indian perspective of ecology and environment is a convocation of concepts, constituting the historical and contemporary environmental consciousness of Indians.

A central percept of green thinking is the belief that current ecological crisis is rooted in anthropocentrism and that Indian mythological texts and socio-cultural traditions suggest a higher value and ethical orientation of integration with nature and its forms. A good environmental sense and status of godliness with elements of spiritualism have been the fundamental feature of India's ancient philosophy.

The doctrine of *Dharma* as an essential constituent of Hinduism perceived the value of maintaining a harmonious relationship with earth, water, and forest.

Rishis and saints considered nature as the mother that sustained their life and that it was an abode of divinity.

The traditions of India as mentioned in *Rigveda*, *Upanishads, Vedanta,* and the *Bhagavada Gita* suggest a cosmic vision of earth on the basis of the fundamental concept of *Vasudhaiva Kutumbakam* (all indeed is *Vasudeva* the eternal reality). Vedic profundity prescribes life with nature, which requires rediscovering our spiritual connection that unites us to the land and that nourishes our souls. The duties towards plants and animals and ecosystem recognize the eco-centric ethics in claiming the fruits of the nature and in managing and maintaining nature.

The common person in India respects and worships rivers, plants, and forests as part of their daily rituals, reflecting a deep-rooted multi-dimensional association with the nature. Ecological sensitivity is well complemented with the cultural and social sensitivity to protect and preserve the nature as part of core culture values. However, in the past few decades of urbanization and industrialization, anthropocentric attitude has caused great damage to natural resources.

Human beings have suffered a lot due to massive afforestation and maladaptive behavioural pattern emerging in urban slums. All areas of earth, both land and sea, have witnessed large-scale damage endangering the community and individual mental health. The pursuit of wellness requires changes in the attitude towards conservation of natural resources possible through pre-environmental interventions at individual, which is great, and institutional levels. In order to promote healthy and harmonious relationships between people and environment, several initiatives are required, and necessary measures at short-term and long-term bases are needed.

Think Box

What is the indigenous conception of ecology? How is it different from what the popular theories propagate?

Key Points:

- Psychological well-being is a central concept and relevant in the areas of research related to epidemiology and its implications for health outcomes
- Ecology also aims to study the invasion and succession among communities and the replacement of one species by another that are more suitable to the changed environment.
- Person–environment analysis provides a useful contribution to understand the impact of contextual and environmental factors as facilitating or impeding factors in well-being.
- Ecopsychology studies the relationship between the well-being of individuals and that of the planet.
- Human and physical component interaction in a synchronized fashion is called behavioural setting.
- Traditional cognitive science approach focus is that behaviour is an outcome of representation-based information processing systems

- The term synomorphy refers to the presence of congruence between topographic features of the setting and behavioural activities taking place in the setting.
- Cultural systems are an ongoing process in which an individual is born. Individuals enter into a world whose meanings are relatively determined through collective actions, and they also try to contribute to its transformation.
- Environmental architecture and aesthetics are positively associated with well-being.
- All social and cultural activities in ancient Indian society suggested a complete harmony of humans with five elements of nature.

Key Terms:

Synomorphy, Circumfacent, Eudaimonic well-being, Life-space, Ecopsychology, *Purusha*, *Lokasamgraha*, *Swadharma*, *sarvodaya*, Ecocentrism

References

Albee, G. W. (1980). A competency model must replace the defect model. In L. A. Bond & J. C. Rosen (Eds.), *Competence and coping during adulthood* (pp. 75–104). University Press of New England.

Baker, R. G. (1968). *Ecological psychology: Concepts and methods for studying the environment of human behavior*. Stanford University Press.

Barker, R., & Grump, P. (1964). *Big school small school*. Stanford University Press.

Bilimoria, P., & Hutchins, P. (1988). On disregards for fruits. Kant and the Gita. In P. Bolimoria and P. Fenner (Eds.), *Religious and comparative thought* (pp. 353–367). Sri Satguru Publications.

Bourdieu, P. (1977). *Outline of a theory of practice*. Cambridge University Press.

Chivian, E., Bernstein, A., Wilson, E. O., Annan, K. A., Secretariat of the Convention on Biological Diversity United Nations Development Programme United Nations Environment Programme & IUCN–The World Conservation Union. (2008). *Sustaining life: how human health depends on biodiversity*. Oxford University Press.

Churich, A., Burgess, J., & Ravenscroft, N. (2011). *Cultural services*. UK National Ecosystems. Assessment, UNEP-WCMC.

Dandekar, R. N. (1979). *Insights into Hinduism*. Ajanta Publications.

DeVries, S., Verheij, R. A., Groenewegen, P. P., & Spreeuwenberg, P. (2003). Natural environments-healthy environments: An exploratory analysis of the relationship between green space and health. *Environment and Planning*, 4(35), 1717–1731.

Geertz, C. (1966). *Agricultural involution: The process of ecological changes in Indonesia*. University of California Press.

Geertz, C. (1973). *The interpretation of cultures: Selected essays*. Basic Books.

Gibson, E. J. (2002). *Perceiving the affordances: A portrait of two psychologists*. Lawrence Erlbaum Associated.

Gibson, J. J. (1979). *The ecological approach to visual perception*. Houghton Mifflin (Reprinted in 1986 by Lawrence Erlbaum Associates).

Grahn, P., & Stigsdotter, U. A. (2003). Landscape planning and stress. *Urban Forestry and Urban Greening, 2*, 1–18.

Jary, D., & Jary, J. (1999). *Dictionary of sociology*. Harper Collins Publishers.

Kaplan, R. (2001). The nature of the view from home. *Journal of Environment and Behaviour*, *35*, 507–542.

Keesing, F., Belden, L. K., Daszak, P., Dobson, A., Harvell, C. D., Holt, R. D., Hutson, P., Jolles, A., James, K. E., Mitchell, C. E., Myers, S. S., Bogich, J., & Ostfeld, R. S. (2010). Impacts of biodiversity on the emergence and transmission of infectious diseases. *Nature*, 468–652.

Kellert, S., & Wilson, E. O. (1995). *The philia hypothesis*. Island Press.

Kuo, F. E., & Sullivans, W. C. (2001). Environment and crime in the inner city – Does vegetation reduce crime. *Journal of Environment and Behaviour, 37*, 343–367.

Leather, P. O., Pyrgas, M., Beale, B., Kweon, B., & Tyler, E. (1998). Plants in the workplace the effects of plant density on productivity, attitudes and perceptions. *Environment and Behaviour*, *30*, 261–282.

Lewin, K. (1931). The conflict between Aristotelian and Galidean models of thought in contemporary psychology. *The Journal of General psychology*, *5*(2), 141–177.

Lewin, K. (1942–44). Problems of research in social psychology. In D. Cartwright (Ed.), *Field theory in social science* (pp. 155–169). Harper & Brothers.

Lewin, K. (1946). Behaviour and development as a function of the total situation. In L. Carmichael (Ed.), *Manual of child psychology* (pp. 791–844). John Wiley & Sons. Inc.

Mc Ginn, C. (1999). *The mysterious flame: Conscious minds in a material world*. Basic Books.

Moore, E. O. (1982). A prison environments effect on health care services demands. *Journal of Environmental Systems, 11*, 17–34.

Ostfeld, R. S., & Keesing, F. (2000). Biodiversity and disease risk: The case of Lyme disease. *Conservation Biology*, *14*, 722–728.

Rigveda (Rigveda) trans in A. T. deNicolas (1976). *Meditations through the Rigveda four-dimensional man*. Nicholas Hay.

Speldwinde, P. C., Cook, A., Davies, P., & Weinstein, P. (2009). A relationship between environmental degradation and mental health in rural western Australia. *Health Place*, *15*, 880–8876.

Sullivans, W. C. (2005). Urban places. Reconnecting with the natural world. In P. Bartlet (Ed.), *Forest Savanna City: Evolutionary landscapes and human functioning* (pp. 237–252). MIT Press.

Tokano, T., Nakamura, K., & Watenabe, M. (2002). Urban residential environments and senior citizens' longevity in megacity areas: The importance of Walkalile green Spaces. *Journal of Epidemiology and Community Health, 56*, 913–918.

Ulrich, R. S. (1984). View through a window may influence recovery from surgery. *Science*, *224*, 420–421.

Ulrich, R. S., Simons, R. F., Lasito, B. D., Florito, E., Miles, M. A., & Zelson, M. (1991). Stress recovery during exposure to natural and urban environments. *Journal of Environmental Psychology*, *11*, 201–230.

4 Work–life and Well-being

Learning Objectives

After reading this chapter, you will be able to understand:

- Psychologically healthy workplaces and well-being
- Occupational health and safety
- Employee empowerment and engagement
- Positive psychology and healthy workplace
- Psychosocial factors and occupational identity
- Respectful workplaces
- Humility and humour
- Religion, spirituality, and work

Introduction

The work ethics acquired greater importance with the onset of modernity and was portrayed as the indicator of true human values. The introduction of large-scale machinery and organizations supporting processes of production led to the emergence of workers, which gave rise to the philosophy to act more and think less.

(David Philip Miller (2019) *The Life and Legend of James Watt*: Collaboration Natural Philosophy and ISBN 13-978-0-8229-558-1 University of Pittsburgh Press, USA)

The scientific temper left nothing to imagination and reflection: nature ought to be conquered. James Watt argued in 1785 that all those whose physical exertion was required to make the inventors ideas turn into flesh, are to be considered in no other light than as mere acting mechanical powers. It is scarcely necessary that they should use their reason.

All the uncontrolled impulses of human desires cast suspicion upon everything people earmarked, which was unschooled as being a part of work–ethics crusade.

DOI: 10.4324/9781003350651-4

For the pioneers of modernity, tradition was a morally disgraceful word, and work ethic stood against the inclinations of the creatures of habit to settle for a crude incomprehensible alien regime.

The concept of work ethic was inspired through preachings from capitalist thinking and moralizing takes to fill young minds, which ultimately resulted in a radical reduction of choice.

In the classical characteristic of modern industrial society, universal employment became the norm, and being out of work appeared as unemployment. To get to work became a pivotal point of individual life, and kind of work performed defined the status of a man in social placement as well as in self-assessment and self-identity.

The type of work and his position in an organization became basic classification criteria of his life standards, defining a man's equals, with whom he could compare himself, to whom he owed respect, and from whom he was entitled to expect or demand deference. The type of work coloured the totality of lifelong activities including his identity, social life, and norms of daily existence. It would be reasonable to assume that work has become the main orientation influencing all other life pursuits and social ordering. In the modern industrial society, major percentage of waking time is taken up by work which sets in the habits of obedience to norms and disciplined behaviour an essential feature in the perpetuation of an orderly society. The scientific management principle advocated by Fredrick Winslow Taylor was another landmark push in the strengthening of work ethics movement.

(Frederick Winslaw Tylor (2010) *The Principles of Scientific Management* originally published (1911) ISBN-978–1.61640–986–9.)

The transformation of individuals to consumers became possible by linking together individual motives to systematic production activities and related identity work of self-construction. Actual consumption process is a thoroughly individual, solitary, and lonely activity, which is satisfied by whipping up a desire which is always private.

The image of 'good life' and work mediated through income and money gradually acquired prime significance in the society with the characteristics of saving, investing, and hoarding as its contributors.

The use of aesthetics to strengthen the work ethic contributes to the emergence of more and more human wants and desires.

Certain jobs became more sought after than the others with their capacity to enable the employees to afford an expensive lifestyle.

People spend years to get certain jobs to get the high status being bestowed on them and for intoxicating sensation of powers they offer.

Certain professions are considered to be elevated while others are known as livelihood-securing occupations. The aesthetic value attached to jobs further divided them into the categories of investing (adventure, excitement, and power) and boring (repetitive monotonous, allowing no power) and getting the job successfully became the core-axis of human activity. With the growing importance of work ethics, employees' and employer's relations produce a complex spectrum of rational and irrational negotiation.

This led to sizeable increase in the number of vocation-hungry aspirants ready to do anything or everything for achieving such aesthetically portrayed professions. Despite a number of laws regulating the hiring of employees, blatant violations occur in course of assigning central positions in the organizations of which some are visible and some are invisible tactics.

Opportunities/Potential/Selection

The phenomenon of poverty and direct physical threat from hunger also resulted into a lopsided use of discretion while granting jobs.

The social–psychological effects of unemployment in a consumer society are particularly painful to people out of work.

Boredom has no space in the dictionary of a consumer society through it is an essential human emotion. Jobs and money earned are treated as medicines against boredom, which set no limits on their achievements, and sky is the limit of consumer dreams. Robert Reich suggested that there are four categories of employees found in the labour market. The first category is of 'symbol manipulators' – inventors, advertisers, and merchandizers of ideas. The second category involves educators of all fields and levels active in the reproduction of employable labour (i.e. labour as commodity-fit to be bought and consumed). The third category comprises people hired for 'personal services rendered mostly top other people in their capacity of consumers' – a large contingent of sellers of products and prompters of the desire to buy them. The fourth category involves 'routine labourers' attached to traditional assembly lines and their 'new and improved' versions in the form of automated electronic appliances – for example checkout points in the malls.

(Reich, Robert B. (1992) *The Work of Nations*. Vintage Books, a division of Random House Inc. New York. ISBN-13–978–0679736158)

In various types of work, bright and dark approaches were adopted to handle the assigned tasks and their supervision by the employees. The people developed and devoted unquestioned commitment to their jobs at the cost of ignoring the psychological demands of the family. In varying degrees, majority of the people working in various organizations experience disorientation in the work–life balance. Separating the boundaries of work and life is extremely difficult, which eventually gives rise to a variety of problems. In most of the work situations, the lines dividing the personal and professional are blurred by erratic conditions of employment and rapidly increasing urban ghettoes that present a situation of risk-ridden life, and maintaining the work–life balance is a big challenge for the working population.

The consequences of this imbalance are in some respects harmful and in some respects disastrous to the well-being of individuals.

The growing importance of jobs and a strong preference for government jobs owing to the stability factor make certain jobs more sought after than others. People spend years doing hard work in India to get a place in the government jobs, particularly civil services. High rates of unemployment in India among youth is a major social problem. India faces a pressing challenge of unemployment among youth; particularly in the age brackets of 15–19 and 20–24 years, it is extremely high among both males and females. The jobs in India come with strenuous efforts to be applied both in government and private sectors. The earnings received by the jobs give the youth a stability factor and as a bread-earner of the family, which come at a price in many situations. The exploitation by the employers is a rampant practice, and it is both visible and implicit in nature. In order to secure the livelihood of the family in a collectivistic culture, the exploitation is a common practice as leaving a job and getting another job easily are almost impossible for many. A lot of work-related harassments, exploitation, and even sexual harassments are often reported in media, and they go unreported in many situations. People committing suicide and facing the discrimination at the workplace are also Indian social realities. Such types of situations compel people to continue with the jobs despite facing blatant violations of dignity as they feel themselves caught in a paradox: If they leave a job, they can't sustain the family, and if they continue with the job, they experience a psychological burden.

The organizations in which people work are guided by the government rules and regulations of labour laws and working conditions. But in reality, the leave rules and service conditions regarding time durations and other policies are not fulfilled in letter and spirit in many situations.

The prevailing circumstances of working conditions for a majority of our population are far from being satisfactory. The dissatisfaction resulting from professional life situations extends to family life, leading to harmful psycho-social outcomes.

Work–life balance conflict is a major problem that societies in the developed and underdeveloped worlds are facing with increased consumerism and materialism. It affects the lives of the people who are discriminated, which further affects the wellness of their families.

Some of the factors are the result of structural inequalities and factors related to inadequate treatment or maltreatment from psychological points of view.

It is majorly a result of constructed environment which can be improved through the recognition of this problem and subsequent steps to repair and improve its functioning. The role of psychologically healthy workplaces, the growing role of positive psychology in the improvement of work–life balance, and role of architecture in developing respectful workplaces have been discussed in subsequent sub-sections. Indian perspective of work and several dimensions of enlightened understanding can become a path-breaking paradigm to improve the balance.

The notion of work–life balance has become a subject of intense interest among scholars and researchers due to the increasing demands of official work and household work and with the resultant implications on work–life balance. The concept of work–life balance is considered crucial as both contributors to this process, namely individuals and the organizations, can benefit with greater harmony and increased productivity. Employees' positive engagements with the work leads to good mental health, whereas a lack of satisfaction and motivation among them leads to higher stress levels.

The well-being of employee both physically and mentally affects their motivation, job satisfaction, and subjective well-being. Work-family conflicts are a substantial source of conflicts, and gender role expectations impact the perceptions regarding work and family roles.

The equilibrium between family and professional life can improve the quality of life and bring satisfaction. The concept of work can be considered as activities of paid employment and other work done for an employer. The notion of 'life' is not related to work, and it can be broken down into free time used in doing leisure activities and spending time with family (Lawson et al., 2013).

The concept of work–life balance relates to time-sharing ratio between work and family. When there is an imbalance between work and family, whether too much owing to work or too much owing to family matters, stress and negative work attitudes can occur, and these can lead to burnout (Lawson et al., 2013).

In the work of Grzywacz and Carlson (2007), work–life balance is described as the achievement of role-related expectations exchanged and shared between people and their role-related partners in the domain of work and family.

Greenhaus and Allen (2010) described work–life balance as the degree to which the effectiveness and satisfaction experienced by a person in terms of his work and family roles are synchronized to his role priorities of life at certain points in time.

The sense of achievement, enjoyment, and pleasure is indicative of positive affective experiences. The individuals having satisfying work–life balance experience happiness which is a vital resource to handle difficult situations.

Work–life balance implicates the attitudes, behaviours, and well-being of employees as well as the effectiveness of the organizations (Au & Ahmed, 2014). The lack of ability to balance with respect to work requirements and personal needs results into stressful situations with implications on mental health.

Psychologically Healthy Workplaces and Well-being

The concept of healthy workplace evolved from the contributions of various disciplines which include physical environment, health promotion, psychosocial environment, occupational health, employee empowerment, engagement, positive psychology, and related constructs.

Workplace as a health resource in the context of physical environment aims at eliminating hazards such as noise pollution, air pollution, poor ergonomic designs, machine safety aspects, and lighting and temperature conditions in physical environment. Many of these factors alone or in combination have the potential to cause stress, and if they are managed well they have the potential to alleviate stress. Work-related health difficulties are also caused by lifestyle problems. Smoking and alcohol consumption are associated with high-risk health problems. Health promotion programmes related to nutrition well-being aimed at improving the overall health of employees can minimize health risks. There are several categories of workplace stressors including work-overload, role conflict, and job dissatisfaction, which are a result of the maladjustment of psycho-social factors.

When investigating the relationship between organizational factor and employee well-being, researches tend to focus on negative effects of workplaces while other researches focus upon factors enhancing well-being.

Kelloway and Day (2005) presented a psychologically healthy workplace model which comprised a combination of psycho-social and physical factors as important components of this process.

This model incorporates cultural aspects, employee involvement, and psychologically safe environment with the encouragement of positive work–life balance.

The holistic approach of healthy workplaces is considered to be a consequence of interactions between individual, organizational, and societal outcomes.

The Stimulating Health Practice Effectiveness (SHAPE) framework is a model of psychologically healthy workplace, identifying categories of healthy workplace practices, depicting the relationships among these categories, and depicting the organizational context in which they are implemented (Grawitch et al., 2006).

Occupational Health and Safety

Occupational health and safety practices enhance the employees' well-being and protect them from safety hazards at work. The goal of occupational health and safety include consistent efforts at promoting and maintaining physical, mental, and social well-being in all occupations.

Organizational health factors are guided by individual factors, work context, and organizational factors shaping the performance at various activities. As regards the individual factors, the aspects of personality, interests, education, training, and experience are considered to be important.

Behavioural modification interventions based upon the principles of recognition, rewards, motivation, and incentives are used to reinforce positive behaviour outcomes. Mullen and Kelloway (2009) designed an intervention program which emphasized safety-specific transformational leadership based on the principle of social learning theory.

According to goal-setting theory (Locke & Lotham, 1990) specific committed, difficult goals consistently lead to better performance as these goals direct employees' attention and influence their motivation.

Similarly, a set of features related to hazard control and safety are adopted which can prevent the possible hazards. Organizational support is the development of mechanisms through which workers value their own contributions and are concerned about their well-being.

Employee Empowerment and Engagement

In the context of work–life balance, empowerment is thought of as an individual's shift in the learning approaches through the process of organizational changes and changes in the attitude towards work.

The idea of employee empowerment is based on the principle that providing employees with the resource's authority, opportunity, requisite motivation, and freedom to do their work as well as providing responsibility of their actions will make them happier. In the contemporary dynamic business environments, organizational commitment and job satisfaction of the employees are considered to be useful which can reinforce the feelings of belongingness, intrinsic motivation, and improved prospects of career development.

Empowerment reflects the set of cognitions perceived by the people about their work environments. An empowered team is characterized by their openness to learn, unlearn, relearn, and willingness to share and co-operate with each other.

Empowerment is a fundamental aspect which leads to organizational success through employee performance. Empowerment is a multidimensional concept which includes competence mapping and ability for self-determination.

Components of work–life quality such as equality, opportunities for independence, self-control, and social cohesion in the work organization strongly contribute to the psychological empowerment.

Empowerment is a psychological belief in the individuals. Confidence in themselves or self-confidence leads to higher levels of performance in the organization. Employees' empowerment is a practice which allows workers to make judgements and decisions impacting their professional work environment.

Job control is also considered to be an important aspect of the empowerment process. Job control comprises two dimensions, namely skill discretion (high skill level, need to learn new things, creativity) and decision authority (freedom in how to work). There have been positive correlations between high job control and coping mechanisms due to its capacity as enabling psychological resource.

Positive Psychology and Healthy Workplace

Positive psychology advocates exploring people's strengths relying on positive resources in individuals and its environments.

The significance of work in well-being is guided by factors of identity, opportunities for social interaction, purpose, engaging challenges, and possibilities for status advancement with better avenues for income. According to Clifton and Harter (2003), there are three stages in the strength-based approach to gainful employment. The first stage is the identification of talents, which involves increasing the employee's awareness of his/her own natural or learned talents. The second stage is the integration of the talents into the employee's self-image, where the person learns to define him/herself according to these talents. The third stage is the actual behavioural change, in which the individual learns to attribute any successes to his or her special talents. There are various types of capitals that people assign importance to, and these are economic, human, social, and psychological capitals.

Positive psychology perspective assigns highest importance to positive psychological capital which comprises hope, efficacy, resilience, and optimism (HERO).

The concept of positive psychological capital (PSY-Cap) comprising the traits of hope, optimism, efficacy, and resilience is considered to be an asset in the workplace. Psychoneuroimmunology (PNI) is the scientific study of bidirectional communication between the brain and immune system, and it is grounded in a fundamental health perspective linking mind and body. Efficacy of our immune system functioning prevents the emerging stress through the release of certain hormones good for our physical health. People with high scores on PSY-cap efficacy can be protected from adverse health effects up to a certain level.

PSY-cap efficacy factors are a result of an outcome of multiple antecedents that are subjective and objective in nature. The interpersonal factors at work guided by interactions and relationships in an organization are an important contribution for individuals' well-being.

Growth goals are an important concept of positive psychology perspective which aims at a desire for personal development over time. Growth goals are more specifically focused at desire for a personally meaningful and progressive process overtimes. Contribution of certain growth goal theorists such as William James, Willam McDougall, Kurt Lewin, Henry Murray, Abraham Maslaw, Edward Decis Richard Ryan's, Jean Piageat, John Nicholls, Carol Dweck, and Semyour Epstein can be highlighted. People's long-term goals seldom have a singular perspective, but the term personally meaningful is often guided a lot by work – identity factors. Agentic growth goals involve growth which include striving towards greater degrees of mastering the humanistic skills or conditions.

Psychosocial Factors and Occupational Identity

Occupational identity is considered to be fluid, dynamic, and developmental in nature.

Occupational identity refers to an individual's positive assessment of the occupation he is engaged in, and it indicates the importance of occupational role to the individual's identity. Occupations are considered integral to one's identity, and they reflect a person's goals and interest in life. The process of matured identity is achieved through occupational routes and major means to communicate one's identity. There is a strong familial, social, and cultural orientation towards finding a good work across the cultures. Vondracek and Skorikov (1997) identified a significant positive correlation between occupational exploration and vocational, identity achievement. Nauta (2012) found that participants' vocational identity was associated with career interest agreement with their parents, and Sang et al. (2016) reported that participants in occupational exploration status also experienced low inter-parental conflict. Occupational identity is also associated with psychological factors of locus of control and self-esteem. Some of the relevant empirical studies in this field also suggest that family functioning, cohesion, and expressiveness are positively correlated with vocational identity.

It is widely prevalent in the studies that occupational identity plays a major role in an individual's identity which is guided by mastery, interest, social, and economic and cultural factors.

Respectful Workplaces

Many studies indicate that subtle cues in our physical environment significantly influence our creative abilities. The guiding principle of this approach further reinforces the view that creating a physical environment that puts people feel relaxed and safe will get the creative ideas properly flowing. The right working environment with adequate colours, lighting, and sounds can stimulate an environment for creativity and innovation.

Some of the aspects of our social environment like judging, surveillance, being always monitored are some of the constraining factors which may undermine the growth of creativity. Respectful organizations and its leaders create more positive, engaging, and transparent workplaces. Respectful workplace is one where acts of professionalism, integrity, trust, fairness, openness, understanding, and dissent are the norm. There is a dramatic shift in workplace cultures where people working in an organization feel they are the priority at the workplace.

Respect as Resource

From an evolutionary perspective, group membership was essential for surviving in the wilderness or contending with a lawless world (Buss, 1991). From this perspective, the feeling of loneliness serves as a practical function of encouraging people to cultivate friendship (Cacioppo et al., 2006). Our social interactions and maintaining fulfilling social relations contribute positively to the well-being.

Respectful interaction conveys a sense of psychological safety, defined as employees' confidence that participation in workplace interactions will sustain their self-esteem (Edmondson, 1999).

In the contemporary world scenario, one can find several examples why players, organizational heads, and senior leaders in the political parties leave their prestigious assignments on the grounds of lack of respect. Throughout our society right from the children demanding more respect from parents, customers demanding more respect from the sellers, students demanding more respect from the teachers, officials demanding more respect from their bosses, to political party workers demanding more respect from the top leadership, almost all indicate an ever-growing demand for respect and social approval.

Respect is a primary motive assigned why people leave or join certain organizations. Respect acts as a signal that one belongs to an organization and has positive reputation working in an organization.

People working in various organizations seek respectful treatment by the team members and in particular respectful treatment by the leaders or authorities. What is the factor that people consistently look forward to, working in an organization?

Researches indicate procedural fairness and being recognized as an important member in the state of affairs of an organization work as significant contributors to the sense of inclusion, and people are very attentive towards any type of relational information from other members of a group. Several lines of research point to the conclusion that people are social beings in that they use their relationships with other individuals or groups to define their social self (Aron & Aron, 1986). The importance and pervasiveness of this need to belong have been shown by research demonstrating that a lack of positive social relationships has detrimental effects on the physical, cognitive, and behavioural levels (Baumister & Leary, 1995).

Think Box

Why people at the top positions quit without having any official compulsions to do so?

The respected as a means can be used to satisfy needs that help us to evaluate our standing within the group or community that one is a member. People in organizations and work places care about respect because it conveys about others' valuations of their worth as individuals.

Respect culture can act as a gatekeeper of the moral community and seen as a value that we strive for regardless of any individual or instrumental benefits. This idea aligns well with Immanuel Kant and his categorical imperative (Hill, 2000, p. 39), which holds that moral behaviour is an end in itself because of 'a rational moral requirement for everyone that is not based or conditional on its serving one's contingent personal ends'.

The self is a multifaceted and dynamic structure with people having distinct selves involving goals, values, and beliefs.

The type of self that is more active than other selves is also known as working self-concept.

Respect serves as a fundamental pillar for building a moral organization.

The popular notion of work success is measured by income or annual packages, but there are numerous dimensions which are at play in maintaining the synergy of organizational members. Continuity of purpose is one of the most important components of happiness in the long run, and for most of the people this comes chiefly through respectful work.

The habit of viewing success in life as a whole is an essential part both of wisdom and of true morality, and respect is one of the precious values which ought to be encouraged in the workplace.

I don't doubt that many people undertake work for livelihood since starvation is too serious an alternative, but, given a chance, where it is possible to do work with respect to a person's constructive impulses he will certainly opt for it. Without self-respect, genuine happiness is scarcely possible.

A person who is ashamed of his work can hardly achieve self-respect.

Mismatch of Mutual Respect

Work-place communities have high job demands and certain kind of resource limitations, excess of which may result in burnout. Sometimes, the boundaries of work shift from professional to personal domains of employees. Violations of implicit and explicit rules of professional civility guided by legitimate tasks criteria take place with an urgency of unexpected contextual factors' emergence. In the recent situation of COVID pandemic, hospital staff including doctors, nurses, and para-medics working overtime and trying to manage the emotional expectations of patients, the hospital administration, and government functionary led to burn out among them.

Even the courts in India have taken several suo-motto-cognizance of the pandemic handling, issuing instructions to the government and hospital administration. This kind of excessive burden results in mistreatment of the people, resulting into intense emotional burden affecting their quality performance.

A psychologically safe environment is almost impossible in such an environment of distress. It is no wonder that blame game erupts in such situations, and a repeated imposition of power over other persons and agencies creates a problematic scenario. Researchers have found a direct relationship between increased job stress and an increased likelihood of engaging in incivility (Roberts et al., 2011).

Job Stress

Behaving in an uncivil manner is often attributed to job stress and role stress at work, but this can't be antecedent factors for an individual engaging in mistreatment. Blau and Anderson (2005) used a 4-year longitudinal study and found employees who experienced work exhaustion were more likely to instigate incivility later, compared to employees who did not experience work exhaustion.

Organizational Injustice

There are situations where acts of unfairness are retaliated, seeking revenge and mistreatment to the employees in organizations. In a negative work environment, people who experience unprovoked mistreatment are likely to react with counter aggression, leading to a cycle of revenge (Helm et al., 1972).

In the workplace, supervisors have a large amount of control and discretion over distributive, procedural, and interactional justice. There are several instances of favourableness and discrimination adopted on the basis of caste, gender, and regional preferences.

According to social interactionist approach to mistreatment, people engage in aggressive acts as a form of retaliation and manifestation of their power. A regular pattern and culture of incivility generate negative affect which may turn into feelings of fear, sadness, hostility, and guilt among the employees at the workplace.

The process of uncivil social exchange violates the norms of mutual respect leading to an incivility spiral among the workers of an organization.

The negative impact of the culture of mistreatment and unfairness of procedural injustice may have negative consequences for an employee's task performance. Many organizations these days focus upon organizational citizenship behaviours which are extra-role behaviours that support the organization but are not formally recognized in an individual's job description.

Employees who experience incivility and other forms of organizational injustice are also likely to be dissatisfied with their work and commitment.

The aforementioned discussion highlights that a respectful work-place environment occurs through civil social encounters and respect shown among co-workers and supervisors. It is also emphasized that people greatly value a sense of belongingness and a positive environment if the workplace promotes respectful work environment.

Religion, Spirituality, and Work

Religion is a particular type of human activity, and its relationship with divine transcendents that which is greater than us. Religion is also considered as a way of life: the fashioning of distinctive emotions, practices, values, and virtues and a distinctive way of beliefs and thinking. All of us experience the transcendent part of life that takes us being slightly different in our day-to-day activities and strong transcendence that defies the structured ways of thinking and comprehension. In the words of philosopher we find that our world is not just a settled, controllable 'totality' of a clearly understood system but is an 'Infinity' that sometimes goes beyond our human control and understanding. In religious and spiritual traditions, many people experience some kind of ascent and contact with transcendence, and, often returning from such an encounter, they find themselves changed in some ways. As a transcendent, God becomes an object of devotion.

Roof (1998) argues that spirituality encompasses four themes: 1) a source of values and ultimate meaning or purpose beyond the self, including a sense of mystery and self-transcendence; 2) a way of understanding; 3) inner awareness; and 4) personal integration.

Spirituality has a harmonizing capacity that involves our inner unity and connectedness with others to broaden reality.

Ideally, spiritual inclination takes us beyond ordinary daily experience and has a transforming effect on our lives and relationships.

A person having faith in God does not mean that he/she will be a spiritual person. Spirituality is about meaning in life, values, and relationships which involve personal values and connectedness. Spirituality involves one's relation with the sacred as distinct from religion which involves adherence to specific beliefs and practices, though at times it is very hard to separate them. Spirituality also involves orientation to help others and do good work, as well as participate in activities of self-interest. There are people who are spiritual but not guided by major traditions of religious beliefs and rituals.

Niebuhr believed that each of us is finite and thus bound by the laws of nature, but at the same time, we are free and able to transcend our situation: We are 'a unity of finiteness and freedom of involvement in natural processes and transcendence over process' (1996, p. 133).

Francis Bacon (1561–1626) is often identified to be producing the first systematic exposition of the modern scientific method, as well as giving out the most important early modern statement about the relationship among science, metaphysics, and theology. Bacon advocated the social role of science in human life. Bacon also questioned the teleological explanations of the world and preferred inductive method of interpretation to be more suitable.

Kant thought true religion is a moral religion founded on rationality, a 'Pure religion of reason' (1960, p. 140), with theology based entirely upon the moral law.

[Levinas (E) Totality and infinity: An Essay on exteriority (Newed. A Lingis Trans) Pittsburg, PA: Duquense University Press.]

Indian Approaches to Work

A central issue of Hinduism suggests dualism that is essential separation between the physical world of the senses or the body and a spiritual reality that also includes human mind. Indian philosophy is essentially spiritual, and it is a rational synthesis which goes on gathering into itself new conceptions as philosophy progresses.

Indian religion is hardly a dogma but a working hypothesis of human conduct, adapted to different stages of spiritual development. Indian thought stirred the depths of spiritual life synthesizing a perfect harmony between the inward and outward. Philosophy in India became critical and refined its own foundations with the changing times. Indian philosophy seeks to know inner truth and comprehensive character of intellectual life.

Indian philosophy is broadly categorized into six schools of (theistic) Nyaya, Vaisheshika, Samkhya, Yoga, Mimansa, and Vedanta and five major heterodox (nastika) schools of Jain, Buddhist, Ajivika, Ajnana, and Charvaka.

Bhagvad Gita and Work.

Balance-The ***Bhagavad Gita*** is the philosophical basis of popular Hinduism.

Gita's philosophy also derives a lot from *Vedas*, *Upanishads*, Buddhism, and the systems of Samkhya and Yoga. *The Gita* does not recognize any ultimate distinctness of individual souls though it believes in the existence of *uttampurusha* or Supreme Soul. According to *the Gita*, a man bound up with *gunas* is a *jivatma* or individual soul; when freed from them, he transforms into *parmatma* or supreme souls. *The Gita* describes: 'He whose mind is deluded by egoism thinks himself the doer of actions which are wrought by the qualities of prakriti, 'Qualities moves among Qualities"[1] (BG Chapter III 27–28). The concept of 'I am the doer' leads to attachment, and doing something freed from desire for possessiveness is a meaningful way of acting.

The persons while working in an organization when root their pleasures to sense objects, it is more likely that they may face attraction as well repulsions depending upon the outcomes. In this way, working becomes a form of bondage, and it is highly likely that people may fall trap to this vicious cycle.

When people work for the sake of work having no craving for the fruit of actions, actions do not contaminate, and doer feels liberated from the bondage. From *the Gita* perspective, a person who gives up attachment to actions and is free from desires for fruits does not have to depend on the outer world for recognition and is more contentfully engaged in action.

All pairs of opposite human emotions such as joy and grief, success and failure, love and hate can be overcome when the performer of act detaches himself/herself with its ownership. Higher forms of goals can be achieved through prolonged practice of Karmayoga which reveals the light of truth in the due course of time.

The true Karmayogi dedicates every work and action to the God without discrimination and doubt. It is the ignorance of people when they start developing a sense of doership through which they fall prey to delusion.

The Gita recognizes three different paths to attain your goals which are known as *Jnana Marga* (the path of wisdom), *Bhakti Marga* (the path of devotion), and *Karma Marga* (the path of action).

No particular path is inferior or superior to each other, and people can achieve whatever they wish following any of these three paths.

The Gita emphasizes equality of states during pain or pleasure and further points that material gains of positions including power are transient in nature to be mastered by endurance and mental discipline.

People can acquire the power of self-mastery and austere happiness by a struggle with one's own nature and achieving the harmony with the divine.

A sense of divine compassion for controlling the ignorance of struggling mind is required, and the motive of philosophic indifference is quite helpful in this regard.

A perfect equality of emotional calm is needed even when the results are unfavourable. The principle of *Lokasamgraha* unifies individuals with universality of oneness in our attitude. *Lokasamgraha* is the attitude of working for the welfare of others even when a person is in a position of authority.

The *Bhagavad Gita* prescribes a philosophy of attachment and non-attachment to co-exist at the same time. This means people while working may be attached to work consciousness but with the freedom from all stain of the passions.

The state of wordly consciousness and becoming free from its bondage can be achieved through the practice of Rajyoga that helps in conquest of mind movements through control of the breathing or pranayama. The principle of *yogah Karmasu Kaushalam* suggests mastering the lower self by the higher spiritual self, meaning excellence in an action.

In order to conquer the distractions of lower self, one should make himself/herself surrender completely to the divine.

The spiritual traits suggested in the *Bhagavad Gita* leading towards perfection are about perfect equality. We must have none, despise none, and be repelled by none, and this is true acknowledgement of divinity in a common man. In our work–life activities, failure is considered as an end in itself, but according to Gita, failure and success are different stages in the same continuum.

There are so many problems in the organizations, which come through power-centrism, and having more experience should liberate one from self-created status and delve into the endless, eternal happiness.

The understanding which integrates mind, heart, and soul acting in synchronization is the guiding principle which can be applied in modern-day organizations. The adoption of ascetic methods may allow persons to use methods like repeated fostings to control once impulses observing solitary silence.

Work-place conflicts and depression due to the denial of promotions or rewards are major problems in the modern-day organizations. People set materialistic ideals of success and failing to reach them lands them into a state of suffering. For an experienced *sadhaka,* such faltering or clouding is a temporary stage in the long path over and above these immediate appearance of rewards or success.

It is quite possible to have stress dealing with circumstantial ups and downs of outward situations, but *Bhagavad Gita* emphasizes that mental thought to be stilled in the silence of self-existent being.

People can achieve these self-revelations through transformations from lower to upper self with calm, passionless, impersonal, and all-pervading self. Our mind can achieve supreme tranquility when it becomes a witness to the universal within, and our ego dissolves into this impersonal existence. When people work with selfless tranquility and impersonality, their works cease to be theirs, cease to bind, or trouble them with their reactions. The lives of people working for coveted positions in the organizations become miserable, and they work hard to achieve them, but in this process they also surrender many loved things. Hence, they become successful by the law of success, but freedom is contingent upon limitations than the actual freedom. The secret of protection lies in the form of Bhakti or climax attitude of the yoga with the mantra *sarvabhutasthitam yo mam bhajanti ektatvam asthitah sarvatha vartamanoopi yogi mayi vartte* (Chapter 6, Verse 31), whose meaning is whoever loves God in all and his soul founded upon the diving oneness, however, he lives and acts, lives and acts in God. It is imperative to exchange the surface orientation with a deeper faith and vision, which may require constant and sustained efforts. People trying to achieve half-hearted goals are in a state of perpetual misery and discouragement; as and when they achieve their short-term targets, they feel an emptiness in themselves as they feel there is no next goal in sight. But if people keep trying persistently with plenty of patience, despite having failed hundred or thousand times, they will achieve divinity of goals through their actions. All our habits are dependent upon influences from the outside, which obstruct us from becoming a vehicle for the divine. When work is done without personal ego and desires and no personal aim is involved, work acquires the form of bliss.

People are capable of acting according to limitations or being free from limitations, and this fact is transcendental, which lies in the liberation of the souls from the limitations of our natural being.

The normal mind acts according to habitual ways of perceiving emotions and reactions, which is guided by externality and the principle of ego. *Gita* suggests adoption of *sattvic* action when the enlightened personality acts with immutable and tranquil soul unaffected by the eager runnings of our external nature.

Ordinary individuals can also acquire God-like qualities in them by awakening the divinity within them or the greater consciousness, overcoming veils which obscure its progression. A spiritually elevated person should possess divine vision and divine sympathy and see and adore one in all animate and inanimate things, the essence of which is reflected by the Sanskrit phrase: *vasudheva sarvam iti.*

True Godhead is the fulfilment of all relations father, mother, lover, friend and refuge of the soul of every creature.

True spiritual orientation is considered to be free from grief and pleasure, fear and fearlessness, and glory and ingloriousness. Transcendence in the *Bhagavad Gita* is not a negation nor devoid of all relations with the universe, rather it is supreme positive cosmic existence which is immeasurable.

The outward activities, when done with infinite divinity, become luminous, *sattvic*, ethical, and spiritually peace giving. The *Bhagavad Gita* also recognizes the distinctions between being and becoming, but these are not considered to be in opposition but in transformation of temporal to the eternal.

The liberated vision sees the divine *prakrit* in all which can't be perceived by the apparent outward fact of our and others' natures. The liberated eye is capable of seeing with complete love and charity in the heart it welcomes, respects noble action, grandeur of love and self-giving captivating, beauty and harmony and marks out the rising godhead of man. The essence of *purushottama* (foremost amongst all men or supreme being) can be grown in a person through the gradual process of practice, and this practice can be done through meditations which allow the process of renunciation to lead to peace.

The sense of 'I-ness', 'me-ness' and 'we-ness' are constructed categories that often obstruct our spiritual growth and love for all, which should be emphasized from the *Bhagavad Gita* perspective.

The equality of love for all is a subtle way of surrendering one's existence to all pervading eternal calm in the realm of divinity. So many times, people are in a state of dilemma that someone is watching over them, not working in expectations with the organizational goals. In the *Bhagavad Gita*, having a questioning attitude towards one's actions is given the highest importance.

When *prakriti* and *purusha* acts in union, they lead to the supreme egoless personality.

Prakriti shapes the action in us; purusha in us or behind us witnesses, assents, bears, and upholds the action.

Our mental 'I' is only a false reflection of self: it is *prakriti-shakti* (nature power), the universal mother account for all that is done in the universe. The three *gunas* are mentioned in the *Gita*. *Sathvia* attaches to happiness, *rajas* attaches to action, and *tamas* covers up the knowledge and attaches to negligence of error and inaction. All people have these three *gunas* (traits) in them, but they have the predominance of one or the other qualities which determine the character and disposition in an individual.

From *sattva* arises knowledge, from *rajas* greed, and from *tamas* negligence, delusions, and ignorance are obtained (Chapter 14, Verse 17).

The highest form of spiritual consciousness is achieved by doing away with these *gunas,* which is called a state of detached superiority. The *Gita* also suggests the multiplicity of standpoints, and each may be true in its perspective. All actions done by a person and the action of self-giving are considered superior. One should follow *swadharma* (one's own nature) while doing a work, and it will yield better results than the well-performed role of another's nature.

We can summarize the points highlighted in the *Gita* in relation to work–life balance. The chief points are renunciation of desires, attachment, the sense of I-ness and my-ness, and the pursuit of success for material gains. People can elevate themselves from low levels of existence to higher levels of existence through actions with spiritual orientation.

People should prefer doing works according to their own nature, and imitation is not a higher form of action. We all have *gunas* (traits) of *sattwic, rajsik*, and *tamsik* nature, but the *guna* we attach importance to gets dominance in our nature. Spiritual evolution is achieved while doing mundane works, and it may be secured through discipline and sacrifice. Harmony and order of the universe can be achieved by a person with *sattvic* mind. Many of our organizational problems are rooted in ego-conflicts, and *Gita* suggests egoless action. The spiritual joy brings more inner calm and peace, and working becomes a bliss in this fashion.

People working with malicious attitudes are considered to be guided by *tamsik* traits. The *rajsic* doer of action is passionate about work and highly desirous of fruits and consequence.

The *sattvic* doer is free from the attachment of egoism and guided by calm and selfless enthusiasm.

Many problems in the modern-day organizations arise owing to doing actions motivated by personal gains and that may create a false sense of superiority or inferiority, whereas the *Gita* suggests doing selfless actions dictated by the divine spirit within us.

Humility and Humour

Humility is one's ability to acknowledge one's mistakes, imperfections, gaps in knowledge, and tendency to have relatively low self-focus; it also reflects 'forgetting of the self' and an appreciation of the value of even small contributions by others. Humility is related to but is distinct from modesty. The concept of modesty focuses primarily on the individual aspect, and it does not include the 'forgetting of the self' aspect. A narcissist person with an exaggerated sense of self-importance does not care about others. Though several qualities like empathy, accountability, decision-making, risk-taking, and organizational commitment are often focused on, but humility as an important constituent has received less attention in the field of work–life situations. Merriam -Webster dictionary defines the word humility as 'freedom from ride or arrogance'. Humble leadership tends to empower employees, which may result in engagement and innovation.

As rightly said by Mother Teresa 'If you are humble nothing will touch you. Neither praise nor disgrace, because you know what you are'. Being humble at the workplace helps to build trust and facilitate learning which are key aspects of personal and organizational development. There are so many verses in the holy *Quran* which teaches about humility. According to *Quran*, the servants of the most merciful are those who walk upon the earth in humility. It has several quotes relating to the respect to others and not to become arrogant. Servant leadership concept is based upon the premise that the servants have insight to admit of benefitting from the expertise of others. Servant leadership emphasizes the responsibility of a leader to empower the ownership, autonomy, and responsibility of followers by encouraging them to think for themselves. Humility is found to have a relationship with sustainable organizational excellence. Humility has the ability to bind leaders and followers together, and it is about serving something greater than 'me' sense.

Humility is considered a classic virtue which can positively contribute to the work–life wellness.

Humour

The word humour refers to a broad set of phenomena and the cognitive processes involved in the perception of funniness and a personality characteristic having to do with the ability to amuse others and make them laugh. Humour and laughter are universal aspects of evolutionary human experience occurring in all cultures throughout the world.

Humour includes all forms of satire, jokes, comedy, and ridicule. In this sense, humour can be aggressive and hostile, as well as benevolent and philosophical (Ruch, 1996). Humour involves a broad multi-faceted construct which can have both cognitive and emotional elements.

Freud used the concept of humour as a healthy defense mechanism. In this view, a humorous perspective mitigates the negative consequences of interpersonal adversities. There are several studies which indicate the role of humour as a coping strategy. Based on Lazarus and Folkman's (1984) transactional model of stress, humour may be viewed as a form of cognitive appraisal which involves perceiving stressful situations in a more benign, less threatening manner (Kuiper et al., 1993).

According to incongruity theories of humour (e.g. Suls, 1972), which can be traced to the philosophical writings of Kant and Schopenhauer, humour involves bringing together of two normally disparate ideas, concepts, or situations in a surprising or unexpected manner.

The Situational Humour Response Questionnaire (SHRG: Martin & Lefcourt, 1984) defines humour in terms of the frequency with which a person smiles and laughs in a wide variety of life situations.

Humour can be used to improve the work–life wellness. Though there are both forms of adaptive and maladaptive humour styles, potentially fruitful outcomes related to mental health can be achieved with the use of positive humours.

Critical Evaluation

Work–life balance is defined as the need to maintain balance between work and other aspects of life of an individual. The emergence of globalization, 24/7 Internet connectivity, mobility, migration, unemployment, and higher costs of living have posed daunting challenges to the concept of work–life balance. In the contemporary modern period of technology-dominated environment, there have been an increase in the list of burdens that work has on the family as well as life of employees.

The pressure of work on employees has been escalating due to advances in information technology, information overloads, and the pace of rising customer expectations, which can be stressful.

Researches in the area of work–life balance indicate that employee motivation and productivity are low when work/life initiatives are low or absent. People have to have several role-based identities, and each domain of roles has to subscribe to different rules. The rise of information and communication technologies has exerted significant influence on individuals challenging the concept of work–life balance, as individuals work remotely causing familial and cultural disconnect. People working in organizations for their livelihood tend to make up for their absence in one space (home) by attempting to discover more satisfaction at work. People also tend to get involved in the vicious cycle of working more and more for better remuneration and in the process ignore the emotional needs of the families. Whenever people tend to work more and more, the feelings, attitudes, abilities, and practices they gain at work place are easily transferred to the home situation which may be positive or negative. Crossing borders between spaces of home and the workplace more often than not causes conflict in maintaining a harmonious balance. With the accentuation of work-from-home culture, people are connected all the time with e-mails, calls, and organizational occupations even being at home.

The work–life balance of females working in homes and the mental misery involved in women's numerous roles seemingly as unpaid labour, as wife and mothers with the anonymity of their home chores, which is not identified as working, are critical points particularly in the Indian context.

The lack of balance without any defined boundaries of work with young children and family has a significant impact on the emotional well-being of housewives.

It is a least researched topic as to how a mother's psychological well-being is affected by the presence of few children at home, a lack of involvement by the husband and other male members, and, above all, the lack of professional status so much hyped in the society. Striving to manage the workload and taking responsibility for the best interest of children, struggling with feelings of not being a good enough mother, and trying to maintain a balance between sensitivity and social stereotypes of a patriarchal society stereotypes present peculiar, complex challenges for the homemakers. Should not the women doing diverse set of works at home with no fixed time schedules be considered in the bracket of working women or super women who are excellent workers without much support and recognition?

Enough literature is available on masculine discrimination at the workplace, stereotypes of marginalizing women implicitly and explicitly to acquire higher positions in the professional world of work.

But the bigger question still demands an answer to the huge population of women in India working at home.

The female stereotypes are associated with characteristics of nurturance, warmth, and supportiveness, and it is used to force the large number of women not to go out from the four walls of home.

The traditional gender role model has a biosocial and cultural origin in which men are considered to be instrumental and women are considered to be expressive in their roles. Work and family interactions are embedded in the broader cultural, institutional, and economic context in which individuals reside. There is a sharp division of household chores between men and women; works such as cooking, cleaning, and child rearing are considered as feminine, and activities outside home such as earning money and working for some kind of paid work are regarded as being masculine. The case of working women is even more complicated who assume the responsibility of household chores and do some paid work.

There is a huge social undermining of the work done by females for home. It is noteworthy to highlight the ignorance of perception of involvement of females in domestic household chores is hardly recognized. There is no formal mechanisms of appreciation of the commitment given to a household for a lifetime by the traditional gender role in a patriarchal society.

There is hardly any mechanisms adopted for the division of domestic work, owing to cultural and emotional stereotyping of the work by the women. Nietzsche (1998) was one of the first thinkers to recognize the fundamental problem of logocentrism and representation that would inevitably lead to present-day postmodernism. Nietzsche argued about crisis of representation and suggested that no reality can be known or understood without being filtered through linguistic and discursive structures whose independent effects often go unrecognized.

Think Box

Does the definition of working women should also include women who are homemakers?

Therefore, this world of women working at home is an 'open secret' – a 'knowing by not knowing' and still is the fundamental feature of Indian social life.

The problem lies in socially constructed naturalization of this entrapment and oppression to go on without any critical discussion of the topic. Silence on the topic of women's exploitation working at home can't overcome the crisis. It is within the terrain of four walls on which women working at home perform their gendered and 'sexualized identities by conforming to the norms of patriarchy'.

Indian women continue to face countless barriers to enter the labour market. They have to face manifold challenges related to the lack of employment opportunities, safety at the workplace, security of tenure, and lack of harmonizing the emotional social dilemma of raising the children or doing work. A typical mindset exists in Indian society that as their male counterparts start earning, women tend to pull out to give more attention to household activities as ignoring them is also related to stigmatization as being ignorant of stereotyped moral duties. India is a country where less than a quarter of women join the labour force. India has among the lowest rates of female labour force participation compared globally, with only parts of Arab world being lower than India (2017 World Bank Report): in textiles, power-looms, and button stitching sectors, millions of Indian women can lose their jobs in the coming decade due to automation.

A major percentage of Indian women working at home have no chances for career progression and have disrupted health parameters. Ironically, government, community organizations, media, and NGOs promote the rhetoric of men and women as being equal work partners, which is yet to see the light of the day.

Summary

This chapter on work–life balance provides an in-depth understanding of the work ethics concept and the subsequent stages of industrialization. The fundamental requirements of food and shelter are a natural attraction for people joining the work-force. It also deals with dark side of people ignoring their psychological health due to their excessive involvement in work.

The notion of work–life balance is a subject of interest among researchers trying to find the ways to overcome the sufferings due to work overload. Several important aspects of family life and other kinds of health hazards have come to the attention of researchers and scholars. The contextual elements of healthy workplaces and expansion of workplace models have been discussed at length.

It also provides a comprehensive review of how occupational health and safety can be adequately managed to enhance physical, mental, and social well-being of workers.

The concept of employee empowerment and engagement has been discussed to describe how empowerment can be considered an important driver of work engagement and the importance of role of work-engagement in motivating employees.

The phenomenon of and the scientific evidence to support the adage 'money can't buy happiness' are explained with the positive psychology perspective. Positive organizational scholarship and positive organizational behaviour examine the dynamics within organizations that influence employees' well-being at subjective, individual, and institutional levels. Although popularized recently, positive psychology has its roots in the very beginnings of psychology with William James' (1902) research on healthy mindedness and Maslow's (1954) call for the study of positive psychology. The current pioneers of the field of positive psychology are Martin Selingman and Csikszentmihalyi (2000), who described that the aim of this field is to focus on positive qualities.

The sub-topic of respectful workplaces encompasses the positive and negative implications of the workplace environment. Psychologically healthy workplaces have the capacity to contribute resource application of the employees. At the same time, incivility and other forms of maltreatment prevalent at the workplace result in stress and dissatisfaction among its employees.

The spiritual dimensions of workplace and its implication for well-being have been discussed in detail. The *Bhagavad Gita* perspective explains seemingly antagonistic perspectives of work and life actually complementing each other.

A lot of emphasis on karma (work) in the *Bhagavad Gita* affirms action as an effective vehicle for purification. The *Gita* also suggests that one must see action in inaction and inaction in action; only then, can one be free of compulsive desire. The *Gita* theory of Karma suggests renouncing the fruit of action, and this way can lead to greater satisfaction. True self is not a theoretical abstraction, but it should empower the person to be egoless and impartial in his actions. The source of myriads of problems in modern-day organizations is based upon superiority and inferiority of success at work with regards to materialistic positions. The teachings of the *Bhagavad Gita* prescribe the goal to transcend I-centred consciousness, and it can be achieved through the knowledge of higher self. De-centring of self-concern is good for the benefit of everyone. The attitude of 'I am not the doer' or of non-ownership can bring freedom for both self and others. It is a comprehensive guide to find spiritual solutions for the work–life wellness. In the last section of critical analysis, the plight of Indian women working of home or doing household work has been highlighted. The dominant theories of academics and researchers paid least attention to the work done by women in their households, excluding them out of work–life balance discussion. This is an area which comprises the majority of Indian women's plight facing multitude of difficulties, having being ignored by the policymakers and the academics. The pycho-social implications of such women need the attention of researchers to gather realistic picture of the problems faced by them. It also addresses the pitfall of ignoring the issue of a large-section of Indian population and antagonisms of work–life balance among them.

The topic of work–life balance has far-reaching implications from short-term to long-term goals of individuals and organizational well-being. Indian society which is still in a transition from tradition to modernity with numerous demographic diversity requires more indigenous concepts and researches to understand and resolve its complexities towards a positive outcome.

> **Think Box**
>
> 1. Reflect upon the traditional Indian conceptualization of work and workplace.
> 2. What role does the workplace environment play in maintaining the mental health?

Key Points:

- All the uncontrolled impulses of human desires cast suspicion upon everything people earmarked, which was unschooled as part of work-ethics crusade.
- In the modern industrial society, major percentage of waking time is taken up by work which sets in the habits of obedience to norms and disciplined behaviour as an essential feature in the perpetuation of an orderly society.
- The use of aesthetics to strengthen the work-ethic contributes to the emergence of more and more human wants and desires.
- The phenomenon of poverty and direct physical threat from hunger also resulted into a lopsided use of discretion while granting jobs.
- The people developed and devoted unquestioned commitment to their jobs at the cost of ignoring the psychological demands of the family.
- The prevailing circumstances of working conditions for a majority of our population are far from being satisfactory.
- The lack of ability to balance work requirements with personal needs results into stressful situations with implications on mental health.
- The holistic approach of healthy workplaces considers that they are a consequence of interaction between individual, organizational, and societal outcomes.
- Interventions of behavioural modifications based upon the principles of recognition, rewards, motivation, and incentives are used to reinforce positive behavioural outcomes.
- Components of work–life quality such as equality, opportunities for independence, self-control, and social cohesion in the work organization strongly contribute to the psychological empowerment.

Key Terms:

Merchandisers, 'Routine labourers', Work–life balance, Psycho-social, Decision authority, Positive psychological capital, psychoneuro-immunology, PSY-cap efficacy, Psychological safety, Extra-role behaviour

References

Aron, A., & Aron, N. E. (1986). *Love as the expansion of self: Understanding attraction and satisfaction*. Hemisphere.

Au, W. C., & Ahmed, P. K. (2014). Sustainable people management through work-life balance: A study of the Malaysian Chinese context'. *Asia, Pacific Journal of Business Administration*, *6*(3), 262–280.

Baumister, R. F., & Leary, M. R. (1995). The need to belong: Desire for interpersonal attachments as a fundamental human motivation. *Psychological Bulletin, 117*, 497–529.

Blau, G., & Anderson, L. (2005). Testing a measure of instigated workplace incivility. *Journal of Occupational and Organizational Psychology, 78*, 596–614.

Buss, D. M. (1991). Evolutionary personality psychology. In M. R. Rosenzweig & L. W. Porter (Eds.), *Annual review of psychology* (Vol. 42, pp. 459–491). Annual Reviews.

Cacioppo, J. T., Hughes, M. E., Waite, L. J., Hawkley, L. C., & Thisted, R. A. (2006). Loneliness as a specific risk factor for depressive symptoms, cross sectional and longitudinal analyses. *Psychology and Aging, 21*, 140–151.

Clifton, D. O., & Harter, J. K. (2003). Strength investments. In K. S. Cameron, J. E. Dutton & R. E. Quinn (Eds.), *Positive organizational scholarship* (pp. 111–121). Berrett-Koehler.

Edmondson, A. (1999). Psychological safety and learning behaviour in work teams. *Administrative Science Quarterly, 44*, 350–383.

Grawitch, M. J., Gottschalk, M., & Munz, D. C. (2006). The path to a healthy workplace: A critical review linking healthy workplace practices, employee well-being, and organizational improvements. *Counselling Psychology Journal: Practice and Research, 58*(3), 129–147.

Greenhaus, G. H., & Allen, T. D. (2010). Work – family balance: A review and extension of the literature. In L. Tetrick & J. C. Quick (Eds.), *Handbook of occupational health psychology* (2nd ed., pp. 165–183). American Psychological Association.

Grzywacz, J., & Carlson, D. (2007). Conceptualizing work – Family balance: Implications for practice and research. *Advances in Developing Human Resources, 9*, 455–471. https://doi.org/10.1177/1523422307305487.

Helm, B., Banoma, T. V., & Tedeschi, J. T. (1972). Reciprocity for harm done. *Journal of Social Psychology, 87*, 89–98.

Hill, T. E. (2000). *Respect, pluralism and justice*. Oxford University Press.

James, W. (1902–1910). *Writings: The varieties of religious experience*. Library of American (1988). ISBN: 13.978-0940450387

Kant, I. (1960). *Religion within the limits of reason alone* (p. 140). Harper & Row (Original work published 1794).

Kelloway, E. K., & Day, A. L. (2005). Building healthy workplaces: What we know so far. *Canadian Journal of Behavioural Science, 37*, 223–235.

Khetan, P. P. (2008a). *The Bhagavad Gita: Chapter-III verse 27–28* (pp. 107–109) Sri Aurobindo Ashram Trust. ISBN: 816510-04-04.

Khetan, P. P. (2008b). *The Bhagavad Gita: Chapter VI verse 31* (p. 235). Sri Aurobindo Ashram Trust. ISBN: 816510-04-04.

Khetan, P. P. (2008c). *The Bhagavad Gita: Chapter 14 verse 17* (p. 472). Sri Aurobindo Ashram Trust. ISBN: 81651-04-04.

Kuiper, N. A., Martin, R. A., & Olinger, L. J. (1993). Coping humor, stress and Cognitive appraisals. *Canadian Journal of Behavioural Sciences, 25*, 81–96.

Lawson, G. M., Duda, J. T., Avants, B. B., Wu, J., & Farah, M. J. (2013a). Associations between children's socioeconomic status and prefrontal cortical thickness. *Developmental Science, 16*, 641–652.

Lawson, K. M., Davis, K. D., Cerouter, A. C., & Neill, J. W. (2013b). Understanding work-family spillover in hotel managers. *International Journal of Hospitality Management, 33*, 273–281.

Lazarus, R., & Folkman, S. (1984). *Stress, appraisal, and coping*. Springer.

Locke, E. A., & Lotham, G. P. (1990). *A theory of goals setting and task performance*. Prentice Hall.

Martin, R. A., & Lefcourt, H. M. (1984). Situational humor response questionnaire: Quantitative measure of sense of humor. *Journal of Personality and Social Psychology, 47*, 145–155.

Maslow, H. (1954). *Motivation and personality*. Harper & Row Publishers.

Mullen, J. E., & Kelloway, E. K. (2009). Safety leadership: A longitudinal study of the effects of transformational leadership on safety outcomes. *Journal of Occupational and Organizational Psychology, 82*, 253–272.

Nauta, M. M. (2012). Are RIASEC, Interest traits: Evidence based on self-other agreement. *Journal of Career Assessment, 20*(4), 426–439.

Niebuhr, R. (1996). *The nature and destiny of man: A Christian interpretation. Volume II: Human destiny* (p. 133). Westminster John Knox Press (Original work published 1943).

Nietzsche, F. (1998). *Beyond good and evil: Prelude to a philosophy of the future* (M. Faber, Trans.). Oxford University Press.

Roberts, S. J., Scherer, L. L., & Bowyer, C. J. (2011). Job stress and incivility: What role does psychological capital play. *Journal of Leadership and Organisational Studies, 18*, 449–458.

Roof, W. C. (1998). Modernity, the religious, and the spiritual. *The ANNALS of the American Academy of Political and Social Science, 558*(1), 211–224.

Ruch, W. (1996). Measurement approaches to the sense of humor introduction and overview. *Human, 5*, 239–250.

Sang, B., Kim, D. W., & Lee, K. H. (2016). Contextual influences on Korean college students vocational identity development. *Asia Pacific Educational Review, 17*(1), 175–184.

Sang, K. J. C., Richards, J., and Marks, A. (2016) Gender and Disability in Male-Dominated Occupations: *A Social Relational Model*. Gender, Work & Organization, 23: 566–581. doi: 10.1111/gwao.12143.

Selingman, M. E. P., & Csikszentmihalyi, M. (2000). Positive psychology: An introduction. *American Psychologist, 55*(1), 5–14.
Suls, J. M. (1972). A two stage model for the appreciation of jokes and cartoons. In J. H. Goldstein & P. E. McGhee (Eds.), *The psychology of humor theoretical perspectives and empirical issues* (pp. 81–100). Academic Press.
Vondracek, F. W., & Skorikov, V. B. (1997). Leisure, School and Work activity preferences and their role in vocational identity development. *The Career Development Quarterly*, *45*(4), 322–340.

5 Culture and Well-being

Learning Objectives

After reading this chapter, you will be able to understand:

- Culture and well-being
- Consumption and well-being
- Indian perspective

Introduction

Cultural knowledge is a shared meaning about the world through which people can engage in meaning-making. Cultural knowledge provides us with the capacity to categorize words, concepts, and classes to make sense of reality, and it provides people the ability to perceive the world as structured information. People use schemata and mental shortcuts to organize to process information and perceptions about the world with the help of previously stored knowledge to make judgments. Cultural knowledge can be declarative, procedural, or evaluative.

Declarative knowledge involves knowledge of the facts and events, and procedural knowledge is the schemata in declarative knowledge. Bourdieu's widely acclaimed concepts of 'habitus' and 'cultural capital' are grounded on the procedural knowledge acquisition (Bourdieu, 1986, pp. 241–258).

Procedural knowledge is broadly categorized into two types: scripts/routines and distributed knowledge. Scripts are cultural algorithms: store knowledge of a 'predetermined stereotyped sequence of actions that defines a well-known situation'.

Even simple scripts are prone to misconceptions and can usually be learned only by doing (Chen, 2004, p. 98). Routines are of two types: individual (performed by a single person) and divisional (done in alignment with others). Divisional knowledge is also known as distributed knowledge (tacit knowledge which is the result of interaction between different knowledge sets). In evaluative aspect, values within the contest of social actors valorize emotion and guide people's action in significant ways.

DOI: 10.4324/9781003350651-5

Values have been distinguished as terminal and instrumental (Rokeach's 1975) as well as general and dominant relevant (Lefkowitz, 2003), which is a psychological tendency to evaluate a particular entity by same degrees of favourableness or unfavourableness. Values are considered to be a force strength influencing the prioritization of choice regarding particular objects.

Norms are crucial components of the evaluative domain which reflects shared values that prescribe and proscribe what we ought to do in a given situation. Norms are central to the functioning of a given social system, guiding the course of human actions.

It is necessary to understand that neglect of the norms aspects while observing a particular group may lead to misleading interpretations of their behaviour. Another significant aspect in the understanding of culture is the role of institutions which are an ensemble of norms containing prescriptive weight.

In Douglas's (1986, p. 92) view,

> Institutions systematically direct individual memory and channel our perceptions into forms compatible with the relations they authorize. They fix processes that are essentially dynamic, they hide their influence and they rouse own emotions to a standardized pitch on standardized issues. They endow themselves with rightness.

The pragmatics of culture signifies power and status differences on the basis of social identities, which also vary according to ascribed statuses of gender, caste, age, and ethnicity.

In all societies, maleness, as Fiske (2010, pp. 951–953) notes, is the deferent gender, the presumption of dominance expressed in verbal and non-verbal terms: 'communication may emphasize male metaphor jargon (sports, military) patronizing speech (girls) on sexual innuendo and joking (p. 951) and the view that this is both natural and morally correct'. Culture is also viewed as a guidance system with its set of rules, norms, and values. Knowledge activation in a given socio-cultural context is guided by availability, accessibility, application, and the degrees of self-regulation about the cultural knowledge. Knowledge activation is seen as a product of the interaction between available knowledge, stimulus, and social context (Anderson et al., 2007, pp. 142–143; Smith, 1998, pp. 408–409). The construct of culture is internalized by the people in the forms of domain-specific knowledge structures.

In fact, group cognition, identity, and emotion are integrated into cultural practice.

It is important to understand that culture and cultural knowledge practices are important ways through which people experience their world, and they have a powerful influence on their behaviour. We can also say that our understanding of culture forms the basis of thoughts and feelings, enabling us to understand the behaviour of the people and its impact on mental health spectrum.

U.S. anthropologist Edward T. Hall (1976) divided cultures according to their ways of communicating: high-context (much of the information is implicit) and low-context cultures (nearly everything is explicit). However, in practice, these two categories overlap with each other as traditional and modern traditions.

Hofstede and others (2010) described six dimensions of culture labelled as:

(1) Power distance, related to the different solutions to the basic problem of inequality.
(2) Uncertainty avoidance: This is related to the levels of stress experienced by people in case of uncertain situations.
(3) Individualism versus collectivism: It is related to the 'I-consciousness' and 'we-consciousness' among the members of a society.
(4) Masculinity versus femininity: It refers to distribution of values between the genders, such as strong qualities for males and sympathy for the females.
(5) Long-term versus short-term orientation: This relates traditions as sacrosanct in the short-term orientation as well as service to others as an important goal and in case of long term orientation traditions are adaptalite to changed circumstances and thrift and perseverance are important goals.
(6) Indulgence versus self-restraint: It is related to the freedom of speech as important in views of indulgence and freedom of speech is not a primary cancer in case of restraint values.

Evolution of Society and Culture

In its earliest stages, the human society thrived on the activities of hunting and gathering as the sole means of sustaining life.

Gradually, herding and horticultural societies came into existence in which people depended mostly on animals and cultivation of some crop for food.

This transition to herding further led to the emergence of an agricultural society. The primary occupation of the agrarian society was to rely primarily on raising crops for food. Wealthy farmers had a larger control over the farms, and a feudal system came into existence forcing peasants to work in lands for masters.

Industrial society emerged with the technological revolution of steam power and gasoline engines permitting the replacement of human and animal power by machines. Industrial society mainly relied upon mechanized production; and problems related to inequality, alienations, exploitation of human labour, and urbanization emerged as challenges for human society.

Post-industrial societies witnessed the growth of multinational corporations, and human labour was transformed to automated production. Daniel Bell (1973) described the transformation of work, information, and communication as 'third technological revolution' after industrialization was based on steam (what he calls the first technological revolution) and the invention of electricity (the second technological revolution). Post-industrial societies were characterized by atomic and solar energy, climate changes, computer-controlled robots, and information technology growth leading to virtual societies. Cultural relativity and Ethnocentrism every custom, belief or action are relevant in the context of culture it occurs. Considering capital punishment is a law in some society, whereas others do not consider it right, both the groups may have sufficient explanations for their viewpoint. Moral judgments are relative in nature, whereas universalist perspective claims that some moral judgments are universally valid.

The rightness or wrongness of a deed is determined by the norms of host culture which may be or may not be rational.

The positive definition of ethnocentrism is 'the point of view that one's own way of life is to be preferred by all others (Herskovits, 1973, p. 21) Ethnocentrism becomes negative when 'one's own group becomes the center of everything and all others' are scaled rated with reference to it (Summer, 1979, p. 13).

The culture differences form the basis of ethnocentrism, and much of apartheid, caste discrimination, and genocide all over the world are examples of negative ethnocentrism.

It is difficult for scientists to decide what is right or wrong because they are capable to predict an outcome which can be measured and verified.

In order to grasp the differences to be relevant in their own context, cultural relativism poses the idea that each culture or ethnic group is to be evaluated on the basis of its own values and norms and not on the basis of those of another culture.

Judgments are based upon the experience which one acquires through enculturation. In other words, our thinking is influenced by social context, and where one stands determines what they see.

The failure to understand or perceive others' point of view leads to attitudinal and behavioural differences between members of different groups.

Several group-level ethnic and casteist clashes ranging for years are based upon the principles of ethnocentrism which may have long-term mental health implications for the conflicting group members' culture and mental health.

The social and cultural background of individuals shape their perceptions and lifestyle preferences, which contribute to certain types of behavioural outcomes. These are several healing and faith systems which use traditional methods to cure mental illness. The significant contributors to the mental illness spectrum can be understood from the racial discrimination, acculturation, bi-cultural self-efficacy, and generational status perspective.

Racial stress

A large number of studies reflect minority population stress related to racial discrimination. Race-related stress refers to the 'race related transactions between individuals as groups and their environment that emerge from the dynamics of racism and that are perceived to threaten well-being'.

The bitter feelings of racism are experienced by individual or groups in course of day-to-day interactions across cultural and institutional domains in the form of explicit/implicit, micro, or macro aggressions, which after a long duration may result in chronic stress. It is very common to hear about discriminations in the school, metro trains, and workplaces which have demoralizing effects on the victims of racism having short-term and long-term effects on well-being. The effect of racism can take place at individual and collective levels.

Collective experience of cultural stress reflects the socio-political and institutional inequalities of stereotypical expression that disadvantages people of certain colour. The effects of racism are insidious (Dovidio & Gaertner, 1986). The promulgations of laws against discrimination on the basis of race have led to the decrease in manifest instances in recent past, but living with the perpetual threat of racism affects the wellness in a person's everyday life, and planning to defend oneself in case of an eventuality poses a lot of mental stress. Therefore, people from the minority race have to expend a considerable amount of psychological, emotional, and physical energy coping with racism-related stress. Racism-related stress has been linked to poorer mental health outcomes (Pak et al., 1991) in Asian American populations.

Acculturative Stress

Acculturations stress are 'those phenomenon which result when groups of individuals having different cultures come into continuous first-hand contact, with subsequent changes in the original cultural patterns of either or both groups' (Redfield et al., 1937, p. 149).

Acculturation is process through which members of a migrant community and their offspring undergo cultural changes across life domains as a result of continuous exposure to the second culture.

Culture-specific stressors are rooted in the acculturation process due to changes in language, communication styles, social norms, and familial gaps in the native culture and the migrant place culture. Acculturation stress can lead to a deterioration in one's mental health status (Williams & Berry, 1991).

Mental health and mental illness are influenced and determined a lot by the socio-cultural factors. Cultural variables of customs, beliefs, norms, and traditions influence the epidemiology, outcome, and treatment of mental illness.

Culture has multiple roles to play in the expression of psychopathological disorder (Tseng, 2001) such as:

1. Pathogenic effects: Culture is a direct causative factor in forming or generating illness.
2. Pathogenic-selective effects: Tendency to select culturally influenced reaction patterns that result in psychopathology.
3. Patho-plastic effects: Culture contributes to modelling or shaping of symptoms.
4. Patho-elaborating effect: Behavioural reactions become exaggerated through cultural reinforcements.
5. Patho-facilitative effects: Cultural factors contribute to frequent occurrence.
6. Patho-reactive effects: Culture influences perception and reaction.

Bicultural Self-efficacy

In this age of globalization and emergence of traditional modern society discourse on multiculturalism and biculturalism or 'dual cultural identity' has gained importance. As compared to mono-culturalists, the bi-culturalists are people who carry the identities of two types of culture together. For example traditional Indian society culture is that of collectivism, strong family bonds, and highly relational society, but the same person going to the United States will have to adopt a culture of individualism and autonomy which is in sharp contrast to the Indian tradition. In the current scenario, a person from India settling in the United States will have to grapple with both sets of norms, namely collectivistic orientation and individualistic orientation. The system of composite self in such situations intricately integrates both aspects of culture favouring a coexistence with apparent conflicts. As long as such biculturalists are able to harmonize the distinct cultural identities, they can achieve a balance in functioning. The problems arises when seemingly opposing cultural needs and drives create adaptational difficulties resulting in conflicts and stress.

Several defence mechanisms are adopted by these biculturalists to achieve balance and adaptation; compartmentalization is a common form of defence mechanism which is adopted by a person to draw a clear distinction between two cultural domains of life without much awareness of conflict on inconsistencies. Culture is not a static construct which changes with every social set up. A paradigm shift in cultural background traits is not transferrable very easily. For example a person from social–spiritual–cultural orientation background may experience conflicts shifting to a professional and materialistic culture. People living in the same society may also experience this bicultural self with the influences of modernization and underlying process of adaptational aspect which may pose a challenging situation resulting in mental health issues.

Generational Status

The term generational status is used to refer the place of birth of an individual or individual's parents. Classical assimilation theory posits that across generations, distribution of educational and economic attainment for immigrant groups converges with those at the native population whereas segmental assimilation perspective rejects the wholesome assimilation and suggests varied educational and economic outcomes within and between immigrant groups. Some of the studies also indicate that under certain circumstances, second-generation children of immigrants receive more favourable outcomes than the children of first-generation immigrants.

The differences in cultural socialization processes across generational status account for, in part, differences in outcomes of cultural engagement and its implications for physical and mental health.

This can be argued on the basis of limited researches in this area that generational status along with other factors may cause cultural stressors to some extent.

Social factors, acculturation factors, bicultural self-efficacy, and generational status play a contributory role leading to adjustment difficulties and mental health implications.

Cultural Sensitivity to Pain

A person's cultural background provides a strong basis to understand, how awe expresses his or her symptoms in a given situation. Pain sensitivity has different meanings for different people, and expression by a person can provide a cue to the psychotherapist for a comprehensive understanding of the pain process.

When there is a mismatch between the perspectives of therapists and the client from a cultural point of view, a tendency to misinterpretation is possible – for example the concept of verbal abuse is a common practice in the rural areas; still, women in large numbers do not complain against this behaviour because of lack of awareness, and they have strong misconceptions that it is a males right to abuse women. Similarly in several tribal belts, pregnant women do the harsh agricultural work and carry woods on their heads, walking miles to reach homes. In normal circumstances, it will be construed as being extreme violations of safety rights as working in hazardous situations may be considered immoral and against human rights, but women there do not protest doing so and keep doing such activities considering it as a part of their duty. Alcoholism and problems related to physical abuse of wives by men after being drunk is a major social problem in rural and tribal India which rarely gets reported to law agencies, and, in case of its being reported, community elders persuade the complainant to withdraw cases.

In urban and educated societies, such problems are considered to be a violation of the rights, and law agencies can initiate strict punishment according to the provisions of IPC and Cr PC (Indian Penal Code and Code of Criminal Procedure).

Pain threshold is the point when the sensation pain is perceived to be distressful requiring some treatment. Different cultures have their own perspective of pain, and terms to describe them vary according to cultures and regions. To describe a pain in English and Hindi languages can have variable interpretations by the clinicians. In North India, people use the term *mitha dard* (sweet pain) which might sound strange to an English-speaking clinician, which is understood as being light pain in the local language. The response to pain is also influenced by masculinity/femininity features and other normative beliefs. As a result, disparities in pain management might occur because patients from different cultures express it differently, and clinicians interpret those problems from their own cultural background causing a gap in the perspectives. Several models of culturally sensitive treatments are used to ascertain the pain in patients from diverse cultures.

A biopsychological perspective by Rollman and Colleagues (2004) recognizes that a large number of factors influence individuals and group differences in behaviour and individual's differ in pain responsiveness with respect to

(1) Monitoring: the extent to which individuals pay attention to internal bodily events
(2) Symptom attribution: the extent to which individuals consider bodily events as being indicative of a dysfunction rather than a normal biological process.
(3) Coping mechanisms: the manner in which individuals cope with negative events, including their dependence on other individuals (such as healthcare providers) and agents (such as analgesics) rather than internal psychological processes.
(4) Somatization: the extent to which negative psychological events and cognitions contribute to increased reports of physical discomfort.

There are also differences in quality of treatment offered due to varying levels of awareness in different sections of the society. The perception of pain and willingness to go for solutions to it are complex mechanisms determined by socio-economic and cultural factors. A major prerequisite for providing culturally sensitive treatment is that clinicians must be aware of the unique cultural context in which they are operating. Other factors influencing treatment may include value awareness, knowledge about stereotypes, and language sensitivity.

Culture and Stress

Traumatic stress disorder was first recognized in the third edition of Diagnostic Statistical Manual of Mental Disorders (DSM III) American Psychiatic

Association. (1980). Diagnostic and statistical manual. Washington, DC: APA Press. Growing conflicts all over the world on regional and ethnic identities have resulted into long-term conflicts which led to the killings of millions and many others becoming victims of non-fatal but symptoms of concern. Psychologists and medical health professionals are receiving diverse categories of patients such as refugees, asylum seekers, immigrants, and victims of armed conflicts and those of natural disasters such as pandemic and earthquake.

Biomedical model often excludes the political and economic dimensional injustice and its impact which may contribute to stress.

People staying in refugee camps or living continuously in warzones have often experienced stress which resembles the post-traumatic stress disorder (PTSD) model.

For instance reports of percentage of PTSD after the occurrence of natural disasters have ranged from 1.5 to 67 percent (Wang et al., 2000) going as high as 99 percent after war or an civil unrest (Raymond, 2000). People suffering from PSTD may feel a heightened sense of danger, and its symptoms fall broadly into four groups of intrusion (flashback of the negative event), avoidance (people), arousal (trouble concentrating), and cognition and mood (trouble in remembering).

PTSD symptoms can vary in intensity in accordance with cultural factors.

The existing evidence among the findings of PTSD prevalence suggests a substantial variability in specific traumatic symptoms across diverse parts of the globe. Marsella et al. (1996) suggested that PTSD prevalence rates may be highest in cultures where avoidance and numbing behaviours are common as such practices may serve to maintain other symptoms (Foa et al., 1989).

Despite the evidence of biological markers in PTSD, components of culture act as perpetuation of post-traumatic events. The role of resilience and protective factors offered by community norms affects the degree of vulnerability towards PTSD symptoms. Another significant aspect supporting the culturally bound syndrome argument is the changing picture of traumatic stress over time from paralysis to hemianesthesia, fatigue, mutism, and intractable trembling to the modern-day PTSD trinity of intrusion, avoidance numbing, and hyperarousal (Herbert & Sageman, 2004).

Social desirability is a strong contribution to the endorsement of symptoms. Power differentials also play an important role in the context of cross-cultural setting for therapeutic relationships. 'Hidden power dynamics and the tacit assumption that Western knowledge trumps local knowledge' can influence how participants choose to answer (Wessels, 1999, p. 275).

Difference of approach regarding stress symptoms is also linked to individualistic and collectivistic orientation differences. The nation of individuality on which the classification of psychopathology is based is relatively unfamiliar in more collectivistic conceptualizations of distress (Bracken et al., 1995).

Cultural differences regarding stress also vary to the extent to which expression of distress is socially sanctioned and reported.

There are factors such as ideological commitment, religious beliefs, and other contextual factors, which can have moderating effects on the perception of stress in a given situation.

The conceptualization and perception of traumatic stress can be strongly influenced by familial, social, and diverse cultural factors. The bio-marker model of PTSD should also consider cross-cultural aspects of traumatic stress factors for a better understanding of this issue.

Consumer Culture and Well-being

Contemporary society is marked by conspicuousness of consumption and affluence, which are influenced by objects of materialism. The human species is no longer surrounded by other human beings, rather there is an ascending curve in favour of acquisition of goods and objects with continuous bombardment of mass-media-medicated advertisements. The natural reflexes of civilization have gone down where new-age modernity has resulted human beings move apart from each other.

Accumulation of profusions is the most striking, which is available in the form of huge departmental stores and shopping malls where an abundance of food, goods, automobiles, and clothing has becomes the primary landscape and the geometrical focus of affluence. Objects are organized in displays where there is too much for everyone, which impose their presence in the minds of consumers directing the purchasing impulse towards networks of objects. The consumers fall in the trap through profusion of commodities created by network of objects. The concept of ambience, thrill, and cool places has emerged where almost everything such as a bar, a dance floor, book store, clothing, or flowers is available for the consumers in a single air-conditioned location. In this neo-culture of consumerizing, products are mingled with grey matter where consumers experience everything around the central concept of ambiance. Majority of these shopping centres adopt a practice of progressive marketing, and a sense of aesthetic work, leisure, nature, and culture is appropriated into the translucent happiness producing anxiety in our real-life situations. The conditioning of needs created in the modern-era person is directed towards objects for satisfaction, which seems to be endless.

There has been sharp boost of demands by the techno-business structure of artificial accelerators, rendering the stabilization of demands impossible.

Needs in the modern era are not based upon authentic gratifications of human desires, but they are based more upon the pressure to emulate the consumerist model. Consumption is largely a result of the system of production in which manufacturers produce the powers of suggestion necessary for the products to be accepted. The logic of apparently arbitrary interchange between objects and needs and unlimited renewal of needs lead to a state of general anxiety.

The advances of affluence and technological developments are fraught with the dangers of environmental destruction. The wide range of industrial and technical activities promoted by the structures of consumption leads to increased levels of air, water, and noise pollution and disruption of natural habitat by the development of new amenities (airports, motorways, highways, etc.).

The cultural model of consumption also promotes psychological and social pressures of mobility, that of status, and competition at all levels causing a lot of burdens in one life for everyone. The major cost of consumer society is produced by a wide range of continual stress and aggression, resulting into a sense of generalized insecurity.

Egalitarian view of well-being

All the political and sociological ideology forces have been applied towards creating the myth of happiness since the emergence of industrial revolution. The myth of well-being proclaims human welfare and equality, which conceal the glaring contradictions of social inequalities.

The complementary myths of well-being are ideologically reinforced in a consumerist culture which lacks social harmonization.

A consumer society through the help of ideological vehicle promotes the myth of secularized well-being, whereas, in fact, it hinders equality hence the well-being.

The sombre myth of continuous progress ignores the large-scale inequalities as temporary dysfunction. The paradoxical affirmation of continued consumerism creates a privileged minority, and available wealth is geared both to structural excess and structural penury. The social structure of privilege maintains domination and organized capability of expert-power, which favour the naive illusion of future affluence for all in order to maintain the hierarchy of power. This system of consumerist culture sustains itself by producing wealth and poverty and by producing many dissatisfactions as satisfactions.

The structural paradox of growth, which thrives on contradictions of wealth and poor, is relegated into the background on the lofty ideals of well-being of all.

It is extremely important and pertinent for social and clinical psychologists to deconstruct the meanings of well-being and poverty embedded within the paradigm of socio-economic structure.

The strategic combination of consumption communication, culture, and affluence adopts the formula for its survival and growth, and it rarely focuses on unemployment, poverty, and underdevelopment except throwing billion dollar programmes to dispel poverty.

There is a growing trend for propagating the concepts of well-being regarding right to health, right to place, right to clean air, right to clean water, and so on. The right to clean air and clear water is a progressive transformation of natural goods into productive forms of commodities, highlighting the contradiction of consumption culture. Educational system has also emerged as a class institution governed by the purchasing power of its users, and not everyone has the same educational opportunities. Knowledge and culture are subtler tools for cultural segregation.

The paradoxical nature of consumerist growth is that it produces goods and needs at the same time but does not produce them at the same rate; the rate of production is guided by industrial productivity, and the rate of production of needs is guided by the logic of social differentiation. The truth of consumption is that it leads to a craving for objects, which is pointless. Consumer behavior is in the ideological discourse on consumptions secures the ordering of signs is both morality and communication system, a structure of exchange.

Think Box

Is the modern education system a great education system equalizer in the society or does it also create class divisions in the society?

Consumer society also perpetuates in the society a learning of social training in consumption. Credit system and credit cards act as access to affluence for a hedonist mentality, which also introduces a regime of the extortion of savings as wage labour power and increase in productivity.

Affluences and consumption are not objective ways of progress, rather they are always lived with myth encouraging masses. The ideologies practices of consumerist culture pose detrimental effects on mental health of individuals. A set of values dominant in consumer culture foster the growth of self-interest and a competition for success at any cost, undermining the welfare of the marginals in the community.

The expansion of advertising and capitalism symbolizes the possession of material goods as integral aspects of self-identity. Culture of consumption perpetuates a number of myths with the help of idealized images of 'good life' and 'body perfect' as two central concepts. Consumer culture can become a 'cage within' as its influences are indirect, and myths are presented as reality which is difficult to achieve for the common citizens. Based on symbolic interacrionism, Solomon (1983) proposed that products are not just consumed for their utilitarian value, but also for their social meaning.

The term 'symbolic purchasing behaviour' has been used to define the act of consuming goods/services for what they signify on the basis of the meaning attached by society (Leigh & Terrance, 1992). The term conspicuous consumption has been used to define the act of purchasing visually conspicuous brands in order to reflect social status and wealth, convey self-image, and boost self-esteem. (Veblen, 1899; Souiden et al., 2011).

Ordinary consumers are influenced to buy socially valued products in order to maintain positive self-image, irrespective of its actual positive value for them. The effect of consumer culture may have short-term and long-term mental health implications.

Cultural relativists emphasize that culture and mental illness are co-constructed, and the phenomenon of mental illness is closely rooted in poverty and helplessness, which is reinforced by socio-political and economic structures.

Think Box

1. Is consumer culture a cage within? Discuss.
2. Consuming culture is a huge contributor to the mental health problems in society. Discuss.

Indian Culture

The understanding of family values, modes of caretaking, upbringing, sexuality, non-verbal emotional exchange, patriarchy, caste system, and parent--child relations must be taken into account as intense emotional exchange issues which finds expression in a culture. The functioning of such factors plays a crucial role in the well-being of individuals in a particular culture. The founder of Indian psycho-analytical association, Grindra Sekhar Bose, in his many communications to Freud emphasized the importance of the maternal relationship, which was the predominant theme in the presenting material, associations, and fantasies of most of his Indian patients. The prolonged infancy period and intimate association with the mother during this period is a central feature of Indian culture.

Individualism and Collectivism

It is argued that the Western mode of psychotherapy emphasizes individualism and promotion of individual self and tends to ignore the collectivist and group orientation of a person. Originally, this concept of individualism and collectivism was presented as opposing characteristics with individualism emphasizing independence and collectivism emphasizing interdependence (Hofstede, 1983). Later studies indicated that dimensions of individualism and collectivism are determined by the situational factors. Individualism and collectivism influence individuals' coping patterns of mental illness.

Individuals in collectivistic societies like India live in a symbiotic relationship with their families seeing themselves as extensions of a collective identity. There may be a possibility for low levels of self-disclosure and differences in emotional orientation owing to the influence of collectivistic cultures.

Culture being a configuration of shared and learned behaviour is composed of values, beliefs, and behaviours (tangible and intangible), which has implications for mental health issues. Cultural traits have many dimensions, and the factors of age, race, ethnicity, family, and many other features do influence how we think, how we respond to distress, and how far comfortable we are in expressing our emotions. Culture influences how individuals manifest symptoms, communicate their symptoms, and cope with the psychological challenges.

There is endless diversity that exists in Indian culture in terms of speech, custom, people, climate, music, and food. India is primarily considered as an agrarian society. The main feature of Indian society in the rural part is the caste system though it is less pronounced in cities. The same caste may have different positions in the social hierarchy for two different regions. At the lowest end, India still has purely tribal groups, many of whom are still living in a food-gathering stage. The uniqueness of Indian village life can be observed till date where one can find bullock carts and huts. One can also observe the presence of weekly markets in which consumer goods and cattle are purchased. The indebtedness of the peasantry in the hands of moneylenders still persists in Indian villages. The lack of medical attention and hygiene highlights the apathy of village life. Village people often worship village deities.

For generations, India had a prevailing tradition of joint family system in which parents, children's spouses, and their offspring lived together.

Migrating number of people from villages to cities in search of jobs in the informal sector comprises a high population. Small nuclear families of agricultural workers migrate from less developed agricultural regions of Bihar, U.P., and Odisha to agriculturally developed states such as Punjab, Haryana, and Gujrat. In most peasant castes, joint family system is a very common phenomenon of Indian society. The agricultural communities have strong joint family system and family mode of work on the farms, which involves all members of the household.

Indian culture is about accommodating plurality of views within a single lifestyle. The people in modern India are caught with a peculiar dilemma to co-exist with the norms of materialistic modern India with Western influence and traditional spiritual India.

The values of faith in Karma and reincarnation, non-violence, and traditions of fasting are part of Indian culture which people use in day-to-day life activities. The concepts of Karma and reincarnation occupy special importance in the context of Indian Culture. It is believed that one's actions in his/her present life determines one's journey to future life-course. The concepts of *Moksha* (salvation) mentions that people may get liberated from the bondage of the cycle of life and death through virtuous actions.

Fulfilling one's duties in four areas the names of which are *Dharma* (religion), *Arth* (money), Kama (lust), and *Moksha* (salvation) ought to be followed by a virtuous person. Linguistic diversity is a unique feature of Indian culture. The oldest detailed exposition of Indian musical theory is formed in *Natyashastra* attributed to Sage Bharata who lived at the beginning of Christian era.

The word *natya* can be translated as 'drama'. Dramas have their general dependence on dance (*nritya*), song (*gita*), and instrumental music (*vadya*). In the form of drama, one can get reflections of the exploits of gods and mirroring of customs of social world.

The dramatic performance is also considered a way to connect with the divine. Drama is considered to be multidimensional and relevant for each category of people such as young people attracted to love, the knowledge seekers attracted to learning, and the passionless attracted to liberation.

Lord Shiva is represented as the dancer-actor par excellence in the form of *Nataraja*. Ancient rules are even practised till date; musical performances take care of time aspects, performed in mornings or afternoons. Much emphasis in Indian culture has been placed on the need for a guru (mentor). In every culture, the clients and clinicians must have the knowledge to describe the idiom of subjective experiences of illness. The guru is a fully illuminated mind who engages in disciplines of Karma (services) and *Jnana* (knowledge), leading to insightful learning for his disciples.

Guru does not teach, rather he teaches the disciple to be free from ignorance, and the conquest of mind is treated as the conquest of world. The physician in Indian tradition is called a *vaidya*. In the traditional Indian society, family counts as a social unit instead of an individual. The progress from darkness to bliss of a *chela* (disciple) is achieved in a dynamic fashion, and two unequals of *guru–chela* end-up becoming the co-equal or even more. The element of complete faith in a guru makes the process of resolution much easier in the psycho-therapy. India is a multi-religious country. The variety of rites and rituals related to *Sanskara* helps in the formation and development of personality. There are childhood *sanskaras* such as *naamkaran* (name-giving), *annaprashan* (first-feeding), and *vidyarambh* (learning the alphabet) performed with salutations to gods and goddesses. Indian society in the spirit of its civilization accorded highest status of goddesses to the women performing the controversial and evil practice of Sati in the past.

The central thought of Jainism known as *ahimsa* (non-violence) meaning abstaining from harming exerts a large influence on Indian psyche.

The philosophy of mindfulness is a central feature of Buddhism, influencing the psycho-therapeutic process in Indian context. Buddhism suggests eightfold path to liberation (*Nirvana*) which includes right vision, right resolve, right speech, right conduct, right means of livelihood, right effort, right mindfulness, and right concentration.

Sufism and Bhakti Movement made valuable contributions to the Indian society and culture. In India *Chishti Silsilah* was founded by Khwaja Muinuddin Chishti who came to India in 1192. He made Ajmer the main center of his teaching, and even today millions of Muslims and Hindus visit his Dargah for the fulfilment of their wishes.

Nizamuddin Auliya (1238–1325) founded *Chishti Silsilah* at Nizamuddin, Delhi, and he was famous for distributing gifts among the needy irrespective of religion. Bhakti Movement took place in Tamil Nadu region between seventh and twelfth century AD. This was reflected in the emotional poems of Narayans (devotees of Vishnu). Bhakti Movement believed in the salvation of all without any distinctions based on caste, creed, or religion.

Ramananda, whose disciples included Hindus and Muslims, had a disciple Kabir, who was a weaver. Kabir believed his god was called by many names such as Rama, Hari, Govinda, Allah, Rahim, or Khuda. A great exponent of Nankana School was Guru Nanak Devji (1469–539) born at Talwarni (Nankana Sahib), and he was a village accountant's son. He preached for an egalitarian social order and emphasized dignified status for women.

Indian culture is one of the most ancient cultures of the world. The values of Indian culture and its socio-cultural traditions play a crucial role in the psychological functioning and well-being of people. The framework of Indian culture has short-term and long-term implications in the behavioural, cognitive, and emotional aspects of an individual's functioning. Inner harmony is the foundation of Indian culture which can be achieved through Karma (action).

Spirituality is the soul of Indian culture, and through spiritual action people can achieve the highest. Mental health is just the tip of the iceberg in this holistic phenomenon of unity of individuals with the divine and variety of psychological problems that can be solved following the rich tradition of Indian culture.

Critical Evaluation

Culture is assigned a fundamental status in the understanding of mental health influencing various dimensions of well-being. Culture is a set of distinctive and normative aspects of a society, which encompasses spiritual, material, intellectual, ways of living, values, and belief systems which can influence how people respond in a variety of situations. Culture is a dynamic concept, and it comprises both implicit and explicit characteristics.

How people perceive comfort or distress in a given situation is guided a lot by the cultural norms.

Human behaviour is a type of social exchange, and the interpretation of the response between two sets of persons is influenced by the cultural norms. Cultural mistrust may cause a lack of willingness to disclose influencing the relationship between the therapists and the clients. The culture of poverty breeds hopelessness, creating behavioural and psychological problems. There are strong interconnections between industrialization, globalization, capitalism, and mental health problems. The culture of poverty involves not just material deprivation, inferior housing, poor sanity environments, and overcrowding, but also related interpersonal and psychological problems of constant feelings of insecurity. Fukuyama (1989) argues that modernity itself has inflicted a world of multiple post-modern visions in which identities (collective or individual) may be threatened when there is a meeting of diverse religions and cultural groups with different values. The role of understanding culture has become very important as many conflicts in the world have cultural differences as its root cause. A thoughtful analysis of culture and conflict may contribute to unearth social and psychological issues related to mental health.

Each culture is considered to be unique in its own right, carrying and conveying sentiments, presumptions, totem, taboo, stigma, history, and healthcare premises which shape the status of mental healthcare in each country. Diverse cultural settings inside a country also do not provide a neat symmetry of characteristics, and different sub-cultural groups allocate priorities of behaviour according to the local norms and traditions. Cultural transitions and acculturation are considered be relevant for the migrants staying in different parts of the world. People in different socio-cultural groups explain the cause of illness according to their belief in psycho-social–cultural realities.

The definitions of mental illness and the definitions of normality and abnormality differ widely across different cultures. The aspects of fears, stigma, and self-disclosure constitute an important part in the understanding of mental health, and their meanings are largely influenced by socio-cultural context. The shared perception of a problem is also influenced by systems of shared ideas and meanings held important in a culture.

The attribution of deviant status and labelling depends upon how a particular society and culture attach symbolic meanings to them. The concept of label is not neutral, and it contains assumptions of negative characteristics associated with it.

Scrambler and Hopkins (1986) distinguished between felt stigma and enacted stigma. Felt stigma involves discrimination solely on the grounds of an implied cultural interiority or unacceptability whereas enacted stigma is the actual discrimination shown to individuals.

An understanding of stigma deviance and labelling impacts the understanding of diagnosis of mental illness across diverse cultural groups.

Medical knowledge as the only valid form of knowledge about health is questioned on the ground that medical facts are also a kind of social creation. Foucault (1976) argued that medical knowledge was a product of historically located process, rather than a reflection of some universal truth.

Several instruments like X-ray, MRT, and stethoscopes serve a purpose to de-humanize patients to render them quiet, passive, and co-operative in their relationship with the medical power of the doctor. The growth of medical technology has reduced the expression role by the patients in the decision-making process, taking doctor–patient communication to the minimalist level.

Values are important aspect guiding the construal of a disorder in the diagnostic process which is diverse in terms of emotion, desire, motivation, and sexuality. Balanced decision-making in the diagnostic process can be arrived at keeping value-based insights into account.

The more effective techniques of linguistic analysis are also associated with the effective diagnostic process of mental health or any other illnesses.

Indian cultural perspective has central features of Karma, reincarnation, non-violence having faith in religion and its rituals, giving divine status to nature and revering trees as gods, rivers as goddesses, giving respect to guru's joint family system, engaging in social services through *bhandara* (community feast), *satsang*, *langar*, providing selfless service to the elderly parents, and having a strong belief in nature and in god as a one integral whole. There are glaring contradictions that have emerged due to consumerism and globalization of Indian society. There may be hardly any culture in the world having 22 languages according to the eighth schedule of Indian constitution. India has also certain classical languages such as Tamil, Sanskrit, Kannada, Telugu, Malayalam, and Adiya. There are several local dialects spoken in specific regions of the country. It is also a land of origin for several religions. The system of caste and sub-caste is an unique feature of the Indian society. India is a pluralistic society characterized by diverse synthesis of culture, religions, and languages. It is very important for the therapists not to use a generalized paradigm to diagnose the problems of diverse population of people having fundamentally different beliefs, values, and culture.

The cultural knowledge of socio-economic inequalities, lack of educational awareness, family issues, and local beliefs can explain the hidden factors determining the mental health issues.

Summary

Mental health problems are a complex mix of subjective and objective experiences of suffering experienced by people and their interpretation by the therapists. The growth of cultural psychiatry questions the universal use of knowledge and technology without giving due sensitivity to cultural contexts. Cultural variables tend to take into account beliefs, attitudes, local ethnography, stereotypes and prejudices, values, and linguistic characteristics which form the shades of grey in the daily lives and conceptions of distress and healing. There are extremely relevant local issues which can help to conceptualize the mental health problems and finding its social exclusion of the immigrants educational exclusion, lack of knowledge of one's values may impact the cultural conflicts and it may have long term implications in the diagnosis and prognosis of mental health issues.

Culturally determined perceptions of what constitutes mental illness also vary from culture to culture. The real challenge for mental health professionals lies in addressing the mental healthcare in diverse cultural contexts and to retain the authentic flavour of how cultures are lived at a local level, not losing their importance simply because these are not codified in some universal categorization models. Racism and racial discriminations contribute to have adverse impacts on mental health on short-term and long-term bases. Race functions as a social construct, and racism-related discrimination has detrimental effects on the well-being and other psychological problems.

Higher prevalence of mental health problems has been found in various ethnic minority groups across the world. The perceived interpersonal racial discrimination is also associated with higher rates of stress.

Majority of the activities done by a person are guided by value preferences. When differences in core values are perceived, the positive effect of resolving a conflict may be counter influenced in order to re-validate and protect their beliefs. The challenge of adopting to a new culture involves mental and emotional dimensions causing stress. The effect of acculturation stress can take place at individual and collective levels of adaptation to a new culture. The process of blending one's native values, customs, and cultural attitudes to a client culture brings adjustment problems leading to mental health problems.

The bicultural self-model is derived from a belief in the individuals' connectedness and interdependence with others. In the contemporary globalized world, growing numbers of individuals internalize more than one culture particularly due to migration. Bicultural individuals move between their two cultural systems causing difficulties in creating a cohesive sense of identity. This incompatibility of two cultural orientations may result in mental health problems. The process of bridging between two quite independent traditions may create psychological tensions and stress.

Generational status refers to the place of birth of an individual or an individuals' parents. The process of assimilation of different ethnic groups at a new place poses identity and relatedness challenges for the first generation of immigrants.

The manifestation of certain mental disorders and their treatment vary according to the norms of a culture. Western societies in general are considered to be more individualistic emphasizing nuclear family, individual success, and pride. Members of such societies do not get much support from their family and community, and they have to depend on institutional support to overcome their problems. On the contrary, in the collectivistic societies like India, joint families and community interdependence with society act as a support to overcome the difficulties. Relevant studies conducted in this field supports the idea that pain relates to factors of beliefs, coping, and tolerance of pain, which varies according to the cultural norms. The relationship between pain and ethnicity is shaped by experience learning and culture. Mistrust about treatment also creates obstacles to pain management. A socio-cultural group's assumption of a pain as normal or serious will determine its course of solutions. Culture influences illness behaviour in a number of ways including classifying something as normal and abnormal, which ultimately impacts the health-seeking behaviour.

The dominant model evaluating the diagnosis of mental health is the bio-medical framework.

The model of diseases assumes disease to be fully accounted for by deviations from the norm of measurable biological (somatic) variables. Bio-medical model ignores the problems related to living, social adjustments, cultural beliefs, existential depression, and various social deviancy conditions as contributors to mental illness. Bio-medical dogma required that all diseases, including mental disease, be conceptualized in terms of derangement of underlying somatic symptoms.

Classical science fostered the notion of the body as a machine, and doctor as an institution was assigned the task of repairing the machine in case of breakdown.

The taxonomy system of bio-medical progressed from symptoms to clusters of symptoms to syndromes and finally to diseases with specific pathogenesis and pathology. There is a need to include a range of factors, leading to the emergence of diseases which may be social, cultural, genetic, and environmental. In bio-medical aspects, aetiology is important, and other factors influencing the mental health are ignored.

Providing an explanation to the patients in strict compartmentalized terms distorts the process of diagnosis hence the prognosis. For example thinking of blood pressure and diabetes as completely somatic and anxiety problems as purely mind-related problems will not be an appropriate way of analysing the illnesses. The professionalization of healthcare industry and therapeutic technology strongly favours approaches to clinical study. Professional dominance of biomedical healthcare professionals has perpetuated prevailing practices, which does not allow the alternative view to emerge which can illuminate and improve mental healthcare.

This is also argued that the medical establishment is not primarily engaged in the disinterested pursuit of knowledge into medical practices, rather it is more engaged in special interest advocacy, pursuing and preserving social power.

It is therefore argued that an exclusive reliance on bio-medicine as the only approach to healthcare needs a serious reconsideration in search of venturing to new sources of wisdom.

Consumerism influences our attitudes and behaviours, infiltrates our entire lives, and creates negative impacts on our mental health. High levels of consumerism are associated with the measures of physical and psychological well-being of individuals. Consumerism is an ideology, and culture which promotes materialistic value orientation affects the well-being. Conspicuous consumerism beliefs create an attitude that goods are a means to happiness, increasing a tendency to have more material possessions. Higher tendency for possessiveness induces envy which can affect the emotional and behavioural dimensions. Environmentalists argue that contemporary cultural patterns of over-consumption present an impending ecological threat to individual, social, global well-being.

Even the world Health Organization (WHO) has drawn its attention to the multidimensional and positive nature of health. In the economically affluent societies, personal status and material wealth have grown substantially, but a large number of people remain deeply unhappy reflecting a paradox of affluence. A culture ascribing too much importance to material affluence does not result into providing meaning, hope, and happiness. The unequal consumption structure with uneven distribution of material and cultural resources damages the individual and collective sense of well-being. From the critical perspective, the concept of well-being also seems to be constructed to complement structural inequality of consumerist culture. In the consumerist culture, people have the illusion of choice, but, from a practical point of view, they have limited choice in consumerism.

Culture of India is too diverse where multiple shades of communities coexist with diversity of faiths and traditions. It is a unique place where thinking men of India visited *ashramas* and *tapovans* or forest hermitages to meditate on the deeper problems of cosmic existence. Indians' love of wisdom for saner pursuits resulted from goals of getting freedom from worry and detachment from the cares of material existence. India has its own characteristic culture in all the vicissitudes through which India has passed, and a certain marked identity is visible.

In the Indian culture, religion is hardly a dogma but a working hypothesis of human conduct based on Karma (action) theory of life. Indian culture realized the value of meditation and looked upon it as the means for the perception of truth. So many transcendental experiences such as telepathy, clairvoyance, and altered states of consciousness are considered neither abnormal nor miraculous. A 'darsana' is a spiritual perception, and its purity is based upon a profound acceptance of experience, realized only when some point of hidden strength within a man, from which he can not only comprehend life, is found through purity of soul.

Renunciation of material desires (*maya*) and personal motives is a part of Indian culture, and the ultimate goal of life is *moksha* (salvation) where a person gives up all his/her desires. Indian culture stimulates highest reverence for nature and sun. Dogs, fire, gods such as earth gods and sky gods along with rivers and forests are worshipped. These traditions of reverence still constitutes the part and parcel of contemporary Indian rituals. Several gurus (seekers of truth) renounce the ease and comfort of wealth to meditate for the eternal, seeking peace of soul through fervour of asceticism. There is a strong presence of *guru–shishya* (teacher–student) tradition prevalent in Indian culture. Service of humanity is considered as the greatest service to the god. Indian culture also suggests plurality of existence integrating into divine unity, and, truly speaking, the essence of all organisms is consciousness. *Ahimsa* (non-violence) is a crucial factor in the principles of Jainism. Time is considered to have no magnitude, and it exists in cyclic nature. For tendency to enjoy suffering and the ways to overcome it, people require detachment from desires. The word *sanskara* is often used in Indian culture indicating moral conduct. The consistent identity of the Western society is represented through the sense of 'I', which is considered as illusion and ignorance in the Indian perspective.

Tapas is a process of preparation for enlightenment leading to spiritual insight. *Dhyana* (meditation) is the steady endeavour to bring mind into harmony with truth. Karma (Compassion), matri (loving-kindness), mudita (cheerfulness), and upaksha (impartiality) are sought after traits in Indian culture. Whatever methods are pursued in our life journey of wisdom, love, or service, once the egoism is destroyed and mind is purified, the individual becomes one with the supreme.

Various viewpoints offered from the Indian cultural perspective suggest that problems of mental health issues need to be perceived from diversity of philosophy and ways of living which can provide significant reflections to understand their dynamics in more meaningful ways. It is not being suggested that Indian psychology perspectives will have all the solutions that humanity is faced with, but this will certainly add substantial reflections to treat human mind and behaviour differently to achieve the goal of supreme state of freedom and meaningfulness.

Think Box

How does culture influence the conceptualization of mental illnesses?

Key Points:

- Declarative knowledge involves knowledge of the facts and events, and procedural knowledge is the schemata in declarative knowledge.
- Norms are crucial components of the evaluative domain, which reflects shared values that prescribe and proscribe what we ought to do in a given situation.
- In fact, group cognition, identity, and emotion are integrated into cultural practice.
- The transition to herding further led to the emergence of an agricultural society.

- The rightness or wrongness of a deed is determined by the norms of host culture which may be or may not be rational.
- Collective experience of cultural stress reflects the socio-political and institutional inequalities of stereotypical expression that disadvantage people of certain colour.
- The term generational status is used to refer the place of birth of an individual or individual's parents.
- Mental health and mental illness are influenced and determined a lot by the socio-cultural factors.
- Individuals in collectivistic societies like India live in a symbiotic relationship with their families seeing themselves as extensions of a collective identity.
- Biomedical model often excludes the political and economic dimensional injustice and its impact which may contribute to stress.

Key Terms:

Consumption, Culture, Well-being, high-context, Masculinity, Power distance, Society, ethnocentrism, Racial stress, Acculturations

References

Anderson, S. M., Moskowitz, G. B., Blair, I. V., & Nosek, B. A. (2007). Automatic thought. In E. T. Higgins & A. W. Kruglanski (Eds.), *Social psychology: Handbook of basic principles* (pp. 138–175). Guilford Press.

Bell, D. (1973). *The coming of post-industrial society.* Heinemann, Google Scholar.

Bourdieu, P. (1986). The forms of capital. In J Richardson (Ed.), *The handbook for theory and research in the society of education* (pp. 241–258). Greenwood.

Bracken, P. J., Gilles, J. E., & Summer Field, D. (1995). Psychological responses to war and atrocity: The limitations of current concepts. *Social Science and Medicine, 50*, 1073–1082.

Chen, X. (2004). Scripts and conceptual change. In P. Li, X. Chen, & H. X. Zhang (Eds.), *Science cognitive and consciousness* (pp. 96–114). Jiangxi People's Press.

Douglas, M. (1986). *How institutions think.* Syracuse University Press.

Dovidio, J. K., & Gaertner, S. L. (Eds.). (1986). *Prejudice, discrimination and racism.* Academic Press.

Fiske, S. T. (2010). Interpersonal stratification. In S. T. Fiske, D. Gilbert, & L. Gardner (Eds.), *Handbook of social psychology* (pp. 941–982). Wiley.

Foa, E. B., Steketee, G., & Rothbaum, B. O. (1989). Behavioral/cognitive conceptualisation of post-traumatic stress disorder. *Behavior Therapy, 20*, 155–176.

Foucault, M. (1976). *History of sexuality.* Translated from the French by Robert Hurley. Pantheon Books. ISBN: 0-394-41775-5

Fukuyama, F. (1989). The end of history? *The National Interest, 16*, 3–18.

Hall, E. T. (1976). *Beyond culture.* Doubleday: Translated to Japanese in 1979 by Keiji Iwata and Yasushi Tani as *Bunka wo koete.* TBS Bruitanika.

Herbert, J. D., & Sageman, M. (2004). 'First Do No Harm' Emerging guidelines for the treatment of posttraumatic reactions. In G. M. Rosen (Ed.), *Post traumatic stress disorder. Issues and controversy* (pp. 213–232). John Wiley & Sons Ltd.

Herskovits, M. J. (1973). *Cultural relativism: Perspectives in cultural pluralism*. Vintage Books.

Hofstede, G. (1983). The cultural relativity of organizational practices and theories. *Journal of International Business Studies, 14*(2), 75–89.

Hofstede, G., Hofsted, G. J., & Miskov, M. (2010). *Cultures and organization: Software of the Mind* (Rev 3rd ed.). MC Graw Hill.

Lefkowitz, J. (2003). Ethics and values in industrial. In *Organizational psychology*. Lawrence Erlbaum Assoc.

Leigh, J., & Terrance, G. (1992). Symbolic interactionism. Its effects on consumer behavior and implications for marketing strategy. *The Journal of Consumer Marketing, 9*, 27–38.

Marsella, A. J., Friedman, M. J., Gerrity, E. T., & Scurfield, R. M. (1996). *Ethnocultural aspects of PTSD. Some choosing thoughts American Psychological Association*. https://*doi.org/10.1037/10555-000*.

Pak, A., Dion, K. L., & Dion, K. K. (1991). Social-psychological correlates of experienced discrimination. Test of double jeopardy hypothesis. *International Journal of Intercultural Relations, 15*, 243–253.

Raymond, N. (2000). The trauma of war in Sierra Leone. *The Lancet, 355*, 2067–2068.

Redfield, R., Linton, R., & Herskovits, M. J. (1937). Memorandum for the study of acculturation. *American Anthropologists, 38*, 149–152.

Rokeach, M. (1975). Long-term value changes initiated by computer feedback. *Journal of Personality and Social Psychology, 32*(3), 467–476.

Rollman, G. B., Abdel-Shaheed, J., Gillespie, J. M., & Jones, K. S. (2004). Does past pain influence current pain: Biological and psychosocial model of Sex differences. *European Journal of Pain, 8*(5), 427–433.

Scrambler, G., & Hopkins, A. (1986). Being epileptic coming to terms with stigma. *Sociology of Health and Illness, 8*, 26–43.

Smith, E. R. (1998). Mental representation and memory. In D. T. Gilbert, S. T. Fiske, & G. Lindzey (Eds.), *The handbook of social psychology* (4th ed., Vol. 1, pp. 391–445). McGraw-Hill.

Solomon, M. R. (1983). The role of products as social stimuli: A symbolic interactionism perspective. *Journal of Consumer Research, 10*(3), 319–329.

Souiden, N. M., Sasd, B., & Pons, F. (2011). A cross-cultural analysis of consumer's conspicuous consumption of branded fashion accessories. *Journal of International Consumer Marketing, 23*(5), 329–343.

Summers, W. G. (1979). *Folkways and mores*. Schocken.

Tseng, W. S. (Ed.). (2001). *Handbook of cultural psychiatry*. Academic Press. ISBN: 9780080525624.

United Nations High Commission an Refugees (UNHCR) (2000–2006). *Global trends: Refugees, asylum seekers, returners, internally displaced and stateless persons*.

Veblen, T. (1899). *The theory of the leisure class: An economic study in the evolution of institutions UNHCR*. Norwood Press.

Wang, X., Gao, L., Shinfuku, N., Zhang, H., Zhao, C., & Shen, Y. (2000). Longitudinal Study of earthquake related PTSD in a randomly selected community sample in North China. *American Journal of Psychiatry, 157*, 1260–1266.
Wessels, M. (1999). Culture, power and community: Intercultural approaches to psychosocial assistance and healing. In K. Nader, N. Dubraw, & B. H. Stamm (Eds.), *Honoring differences: Cultural Issues in the treatment of trauma and loss* (pp. 267–280). Brunner/Mazel.
Williams, C. L., & Berry, J. W. (1991). Primary prevention of acculturative stress among refugees: Application of psychological theory and practice. *American Psychologist, 46*(6), 632–641.

6 Spirituality and Well-being

Learning Objectives

After reading this chapter, you will be able to understand:

- The rational and secular
- Mysticism and spirituality
- Faith, religion, and motivation
- Spirituality and coping
- Gratitude, hope, forgiveness, and well-being
- Indian approaches of well-being
- *Guru–shishya* tradition, Ayurveda, yoga music

Introduction

Spirituality is referred to contrast with materialistic ways of being and to have contact with spirits and psychological phenomenon of transcendence. It is also used to denote the experiential and personal side of our relationship with the sacred.

It is the orientation of a person towards the values which have a purpose beyond the self and a way of discovering inner awareness. Most vision of spirituality also involves contact with the sacred or 'those forces whose dominance over man increases or seems to increase in proportion to man's effort to master them' (Girad, 1977, p. 31, Cf. Roehlkepartain, 2004). Spirituality has a powerful, mysterious quality that can't be reduced to a simple object of study (May, 2004, p. 183).

Spirituality takes people beyond ordinary sense realities, and it has transforming effects on our lives and relationships. The search for meaning in life can also be practised by the people who are nontheist. As compared to religious practices which are guided by strong beliefs and rituals, spiritual practices focus more on natural experiences, personal values, and meanings in life.

Jeringon (2001) offers a thin definition of spirituality as 'the organization (centering) of individual and collective life around dynamic patterns of

DOI: 10.4324/9781003350651-6

meaning, values and relationships that are truste to make life worthwhile (or at least livale) and death meaningful' (p. 418).

Several scholars try to separate religiosity and spirituality as distinct concepts, while others tend to perceive them as being interconnected. It is worth mentioning that scientists also have a strong attraction to this concept of spirituality because they tend to tap universal human qualities related to invariant natural laws which can be discovered through research.

The Rational and Secular

The approach of spirituality focuses more upon human-centred frame of reference and considers human flourishing as a key component to achieve human goals.

The existential approach suggests that the dialectic between nature and freedom is repeated in human situations. The people who are able to stand in balance between the demands of existence and their essence as a free person are considered to be integrated; however, it is difficult to achieve. The awareness of the situation of finitude, lack of meaning, and helplessness head to ontological anxiety, a built-in system in our existence, and it should be accepted. When the people start fleeing from ontological anxiety, it leads to an emergence of irrational fears with inner conflicts called neurotic anxiety. Rogers considered self-estrangement as an incongruence between our true self and societal expectations, which impedes our growth. On the other hand, Tillich argued that estrangement is ultimately built in existence, and we need more than human sources of existence. Prominent theologian Reinold Neibuhr believed that each of us is finite and thus bind by the laws of nature, but at the same time we are free to transcend our situation: we are 'a unity of finiteness and freedom, of involvement in natural processes and transcendence over process' (1966a). This paradox of finiteness and freedom is the occasion not the cause of human problems. This essential homelessness of human spirit is the ground of religion, for the self which stands outside itself, and the world cannot find the meaning of life in itself or the world (1966b).

Freedom has both the sides of being good or evil.

The experience of consciousness is personal to each person, and it is always different from that of others.

The higher stages of consciousness are perceived to be unusual, and people who lack ability to communicate such experiences to others are known to have altered states of consciousness.

Many religious experiences also convey profound emotional states, which become a source of positive emotions.

Mysticism and Spirituality

Mysticism has been strongly associated with religious and spiritual traditions.

William James (1961, pp. 299–300) identified the following as being central features of mystical experience:

- Ineffability: A felt inability to describe the experience.
- Noetic quality: a sense that something fundamental was learned.
- Transiency: the experience lasts for a brief period of time.
- Positivity: a sense that the experience was not under the person's control.

Mystical experiences vary in intensity and generally involve an experience of transcendence beyond normal categories.

A way of life in which mystical states are valued and sought after is known as mysticism (Hood, 2001, p. 155; Vergote, 2003).

One of the important constituents of mystical experience involves changes in attention and flow experiences. According to Maslow, a state similar to mysticism is the peak experience in which emotional reactions include 'a special flavor of wonder, of owe, of reverence of humility or surrender before experience as something great' (Maslow, 1999, p. 98).

James attributed central place to the religions in his theory of religious experience.

He noted that many religious figures were very sensitive and had 'abnormal psychic visitations' as well as a conflicted and melancholic inner life (1961, p. 25). According to his perspective, healthy minded people have a natural sense of happiness and optimism, while a sick-souled person sees life as insecure with real evil. James further argued that the sick-souled individual had not only a more complete but also more conflicted view of the world; as a result, they often struggle with melancholy and philosophical pessimism. In general, religious viewpoint in its true sense is considered to be wanting intimacy with the universe and anti-religious materialism aligned with cynicism. People also acquire the tendency of saintliness which has the inherent advantages of sacrifice, self-surrender, charity, patience, and purity, somewhat similar traits of spirituality.

Most of the empirical studies conducted in the field indicate positive correlation between mystical and religious experiences to lead to better subjective well-being. But in certain situations, mystical experiences could also feed narcissism, and seekers could misunderstand their pathology for higher states of consciousness. Otto believed that each of us had the capacity to develop the 'holy' as a 'category of interpretation and valuation peculiar to the sphere of religion' (1950, p. 5).

American theologian Jonathan Edwards described the question of religious experience as 'What is the nature of true religion? And wherein lie the distinguishing notes of that virtue and holiness that is acceptance in the sight of God' (2004, p. 15). The conclusion of his work was that 'True Religion in great part, consists in Holy affections' (2004, 4.23).

Carl Jung in his theory talked about the crisis of modern man arising owing to ignoring the unconsciousness, irrational side of self, which earlier helped to harmonize conscious and unconscious forces. Jung's important concept for describing spiritual and personal growth was individualism, which means maturational process of reuniting the unconscious materials with the conscious for achieving wholeness by a person. Erikson considered that adult religious rituals were partly related to common, childhood activity called ritualization 'an agreed-upon-interplay between at least two persons who repeat at meaningful intervals and in recurring contexts' (1966, pp. 602, 603). Erikson believed ritualization as relational becomes more complex, as new elements are added during the development, and following this ritualism becomes compulsive and legalistic. Erickson also talked about people's subjective identity and awareness of 'I' or numinous sense of awareness that goes with consciousness.

According to Winnicott, religion does not happen inside or outside of us but in our transitional space, where it is centrally placed to affect all aspects of the self (Winnicott, 1975, p. 96). The space begins to assume religious functions early in life with the formation of a God-object or God-image in the space that can act as a transitional object (Winnicott, 1990, pp. 100–101).

Religious experience is suggested to have two possible universal dimensions: emotional episodes of awe, peace, or tranquility and a feeling of unitary experience. Rituals or activities related to religious activities include fasting, *bhajans*, meditative concentration, and dancing which possess the ability to activate different neurotransmitter systems. There are five categories of excitatory events relevant to religious experiences (D'Aquili & Newberg, 2000).

- Trophotropic, producing a relaxed yet vigilant mental state as in mediation.
- Ergotropic, which produces aroused alertness as in flow states.
- Trophotropic with ergotropic spillover leading to feelings of energy or 'oceanic bliss'.
- Ergotropic with trophotropic spillover as in ecstasy experiences maximal stimulation of both systems leading to the most intense mystical experiences. In their opinion, all kinds of religious experiences involve the operations of a holistic operator (which enables us to see gestalts) which generates a sense of unity and thus of self-transcendence and transformation (D'Aquili & Newberg, 2000).

Conception of Faith

Fowler articulated his theory of faith as an evolving sense of spirit and relatedness to others, which provides meaning and coherence allowing participation in an 'ultimate environment' (1996, p. 21).

According to Fowler, faith is a more fundamental category than religion which involves beliefs, practices, and images that express and inform faith (Fowler & Dell, 2004). In his view, faith also creates triadic relationships between ourselves others and 'shared centers of value and power' (1996,

p. 21). He further argued that some people have multiple centres of value with no centre having many compartmentalized identities and more between these different interests and situations, and such people are called polytheists. Another set of people who have identity unified around a single centre of power are known as henotheists.

Fowler in his description of stages of faith development suggested gradual progression from parental sources to traditions and finally to the stage of self-acceptance and Keonosis or emptying self.

The importance of studying the religiosity-spiritualism continuum gets reinforced with relevant studies related to motivation and its role in coping mechanisms with implications on mental health. It is also relevant to point out that people following religiosity and spiritual practices find significant shifts in their cognitive perspectives.

Religion and Motivation

Religious motivation theory is initially credited to Gordon Allport's concept of intrinsic (I) and extrinsic (E) motivation. According to him, only 10% of church members will qualify for purely I and rest of them may be guided by E connected with prejudice (Allport, 1966; Allport & Ross, 1967, pp. 434–435; Reiss & Havercamp, 1998).

Multivariate belief–motivation theory of religiousness (Schaefer & Gorsuch, 1992) assumes that religious motivation will have important interactions with belief, coping styles, and other important variables such as psychological well-being.

Some of the researches in this field indicate positive relationships between religious motivation and rewards of personal security and social relationships. Daniel Batson described religious motivation as quest that includes (1) a readiness to criticize self and to face complexity or existential questions, (2) perception of doubts as positive and resistance to clear-cut answers or commitment, and 3) openness to change (Batson & Schoenrade, 1991; Batson et al., 1993).

A lot of discussion and debate had emerged on the topic of quest being a type of religious motivation or personality characteristic. But, in general, it has been found to be positively related with openness to experience and low levels of prejudiced behaviour.

Religiosity and spiritual orientation also help in successful aging. Spiritually oriented people often report high levels of life satisfactions, and they can overcome common problems with hope and optimism.

Bereavement or the loss of loved ones can be less painful for the spiritually mature persons.

Religious beliefs develop the acceptance towards death as a natural process, and belief in the actions of divine helps them to cope with the difficulty. Religious beliefs about life after death and the eternal belief in eternity of soul also help in the coping mechanisms.

Spirituality and Coping

Religious and spiritual activities through cognitive and behavioural processes lead to coping behaviour. Coping is triggered as a result of cognitive appraisals or judgements that what we are confronting is stressful, representing (1) a threat of harm or loss as a challenge with a possibility of growth or (2) something beneficial (Folkman & Lazarus, 1985). Coping involves our beliefs about ourselves and the world which can be facilitated or hindered by spiritual beliefs and practices.

These are three types of coping mentioned in the majority of texts which include emotion-focused coping (managing distressing emotions), problem-focused coping (trying to change the situation causing stress), and religious coping (use of religious beliefs and practices to overcome stress).

One of the influential theories related to religion and coping is that of Pargament (1997). For Pargament, coping is the 'continually changing process through which individuals try to understand and deal with significant personal or situational demands in their lives' (1990, p. 198). Religion acts as a fundamental agent to find the connection with sacred, which ultimately improves a sense of meaning, control, intimacy, or support. People having strong faith in religion get more support to overcome the difficulties with the hope and connectivity to the divine. Pargament argues that there are three main styles of religious coping: (1) self-directing coping that acknowledges the presence of sacred but relies on self to solve the problem, (2) deferring coping – in this the responsibility for a problem is deferred to God, and (3) collaborative style, which involves an active partnership between individual and God.

Other prominent coping styles include surrendering to God, which involves active surrender to God in a situation; positive religious coping with a focus on problem-solving with benevolent, loving, and forgiving attitude; and negative religious coping, indicating a spiritual disconnect where God is seen as punishing.

Gratitude and Well-being

From a positive psychology perspective, gratitude is a virtue which impacts the well-being of people. Spiritual and religious activities are highly connected with expressions of gratitude.

Gratitude is a commonly experienced emotion also conceptualized as an attitude, a moral virtue, a personality trait, and a coping response. From a spiritual and religious point of view, God is considered as ultimate giver, and almost all religions promote this belief among its followers. The spiritual quality of gratitude is aptly conveyed by Streng (1989):people recognize that they are connected to each other in a mysterious and miraculous way that is not fully determined by physical forces, but is part of a wider, or transcendent context (p. 5).

From a spiritual perspective, gratitude is considered as a human strength which has moral precursors and consequences. Persons having grateful disposition are good in relational well-being. Among the big five factors of personality, grateful disposition seems to be related most strongly with agreeableness (positivity) and neuroticism (negativity). It is also found through gratitude questionnaires that grateful people report higher levels of positive emotions, life satisfaction, vitality, optimism, and lower levels of depression and stress.

As a social emotion, expressions of gratitude and appreciation are contributors to long-term inter-personal relationships.

Hope and Well-being

'Let me not beg for the stilling of my pain but for the heart to conquer it' (Rabindra Nath Tagore (1861–1941), famous Indian poet and philosopher). Indian perspective of thinking known as *Darsana* constitutes the attempt to integrate theoretical difficulties with practical and transcendental approach. Indian philosophy also suggests that goal of life is to acquire higher levels of consciousness available within a person's awareness.

Every person is considered capable of transforming future course of events by undertaking virtuous actions.

Based on Vedic understanding of Sri Aurobindo, Sarkar described that hopes in the greater life are not illusions: they sing joyfully like Sangsten birds: their bright-hued glimmer is that of a burning fire that has light and force (Sarkar, 2011, p. 94). Vivekananda explains the importance of hope through an old Indian story. There was a great king in ancient India who once asked four questions, of which one was 'what is most wonderful thing in the world?' Hope was the answer. This is the most wonderful thing. Day and nights, we see, people dying around us, and yet we think we shall not die, we never think we shall die, or that we shall suffer. Each man thinks that success will be his, hoping against all hopes, against all odds, against all mathematical reasoning (Vivekananda, 2015).

The *Bhagavad Gita* suggests arriving to hope to achieve liberation and self-realization. It mentions about an inner force of hope which comes from an attitude of humility and not hoping anything from others as it may accentuate dependence of a person. According to the principle of Indian philosophy, we should not hope about getting anything from others, rather hope from within. In the context of non-duality principle, hope and hopelessness, like optimism and pessimism, must not be considered opposites but the two sides of the same coin. Hopeless suffering is sometimes the best way to discover the need for inner-transformation liberation and self-realization, giving birth to a new quality of hope. Religious and spiritual people have higher perceived hopes with religious faith which improve their well-being.

In his seminal book, *The Psychology of Hope*, published in 1994, Synder described hope as a motivational state based on goals, pathways, and agency goal-directed thinking.

Pathways thinking allows people to find routes around obstacles to goals. Agency is somewhat similar to willpower, which refers to the motivation for individuals to sustain their goals. Snyder's colleagues note that pathways and agency thinking are positively correlated, additive, but neither component alone defines hope. There are several situations in which hope as a construct can be used to bring positive outcomes. Several hope programmes such as hope games, pathways, and agency thoughts which can improve hope score across all groups of people.

Depression and negative life events are less intense for those who are hopeful. Researches in this field also indicate hope as a robust predictor of mental health. Hopeful people are more likely to take action during challenging times. In some situations, hope is considered a bedrock of getting out of suicidal mental states.

Forgiveness and Well-being

Forgiveness is the ability to tolerate the offences of others without feeling the need to retaliate. The Sanskrit word for 'forgiveness' is *Ksama* which can be split into two words *Ksa* (to decrease) and *ma* (measure or degree); hence, forgiveness is the ability for not retaliating against the person who has wronged us.

In traditional Indian Philosophy, God is considered as the ocean of compassion (*Karuna Sagara*), a reservoir of loving kindness that exceeds all limitations.

It also suggests surrendering of selfishness (*Kama*), anger (*Krodha*), delusion (*Moha*), hubris (*Mada*), greed (*Lobha*), and jealousy (*Matsarya*) in order to become a graceful person.

There is a famous story about a famous sage Bhrigu who wanted to test the compassion of Vishnu and so he kicked him in the chest while he was sleeping; immediately, Vishnu awoke and realizing what had happened, he began massaging Bhrigu's foot, saying 'my chest is as hard as a diamond, your foot must be hurting – let me massage it for you'. The core belief in reincarnation and the cycles of birth and rebirth is determined by the law of Karma (action), which has implications for the understanding of forgiveness. Forgiveness in Indian philosophy is a broader concept, and it is away towards working in the service of divinity to free oneself from bad Karma.

One who unconditionally forgives also is happy because the anger on the forgiven is exterminated.

Forgiveness as a virtue is also emphasized in Islam and Christianity.

Forgiveness and mental health

Forgiveness has direct and indirect implications for mental health. The direct effect of forgiveness on mental health can be described in terms of unforgiveness, through rumination, and involving the emotions of resentment, bitterness, hatred, hostility, residual anger, and fear (Worthington et al., 2001). There are many ways to address unforgiveness (Worthington & Wade, 1999). Forgiveness involves the contamination or prevention of unforgiveness with strong, positive, love-based emotions (Worthington et al., 2001). The emotions of forgiveness bring physiological changes that may have their effect on mental health and well-being. Forgiveness is likely to promote mental health indirectly through variables such as social support, interpersonal functioning, and health behaviour (Temoshok & Chandra, 2000; Worthington et al., 2001). The mediating variables of social support and interpersonal relations are contributory factors for mental health and well-being. High scores on forgiveness are generally associated with low scores on anxiety and depression. In some of the studies, forgiveness has been seen to have contributed in the treatment of alcoholism and combat-related PTSD (post-traumatic stress disorder).

Enright et al. (1998) provided a list of four broad phases of forgiveness: uncovering, decision, work, and deepening. Uncovering refers to the awareness of the problem and emotional pain following an offence, including anger and insight. Decision includes the realization of need for an alternate resolution. Work includes processes such as reframing, empathy, and acceptance of pain. Deepening includes finding meaning and universality.

Rumination is associated with a variety of mental health outcomes, especially depression (Harrington & Blankenship, 2002).

The process of attribution also plays a crucial role in the relationship between forgiveness and mental wellness.

The ability to forgive is thought to be positively associated with personal control in one's life (Benson, 1992; Hope, 1987) and the restoration of a sense of personal power (McCullough & Worthington, 1994).

The attitude and thinking of forgiving cognitions and behaviours are indicators of better mental health. Whereas failure to forgive is associated with poor mental health. There is a significant agreement among the researchers about the relationship between personality factors and mental health.

The factor of extraversion is positively related with forgiveness, and the factor of neuroticism is negatively related with forgiveness in some studies.

In addition to personality variables, coping style of a person is also known to be a crucial factor predicting the relationship between forgiveness and mental health. Measures of different aspects of forgiveness can be readily identified with personality-coping factors identified by Ferguson (2001), and, therefore, researchers in this area may explore to combine forgiveness with personality and coping variables for future research.

Indian Traditions of Spirituality and Its Contribution to Wellness

The *Guru–Shishya* Tradition and Well-being

The *Guru–Shishya* tradition (lineage) denotes a succession of teachers and disciples in traditional Indian cultures and religions. This tradition of *Guru–Shishya* has been an integral feature of *Upanishads*, Jainism, Sikhism, and Buddhism. All kinds of knowledge and teachings are transmitted from a guru (teacher) to a *shishya* (disciple) through an integral bonding of relationships. This relationship between a guru and a *shishya* is based on devotion, commitment, and obedience of the student, sharing esoteric wisdom.

In this tradition, the transfer of knowledge and wisdom is acquired living with the guru for years, and this knowledge is achieved being in close proximity with the master. The devotion of a disciple towards his guru also engages complete submission to seek spiritual salvation. The oldest reference to the concept of guru is in Hinduism texts. The guru concept has been proposed in Vajrayana Buddhism in which the *tantrick* guru is considered a figure of worship and whose instructions are always revered. In Sikhism, the guru tradition has played a key role since its inception in the fifteenth century and of its holy scripture known as Guru Granth Sahib. In Buddhist tradition, the teacher is regarded as the root of spiritual realization and the basis for showing an insightful path.

In tantrik Buddhism, the guru is perceived as the way itself. Guru is not a person but a state of mind who possesses the qualities of Bodhisattva.

In the *Upanishads*, *Chandogya Upanishad* suggested that insights leading to self-knowledge can be attained only through a guru. Other *Upanishads* such as *Katha Upanishad* and *Taittiriya Upanishad* also highlight the importance of guru in the process of discovering and experiencing the truth. *Shvetashvatara Upanishad* equates the need of reverence and devotion for guru to be the same as God.

Advaita Vedanta traces its roots to *Upanishads* and accepts *purushartha* and any four goals of human life as *Dharma* (duties), *Artha* (means to sustain life), *Kama* (pleasure), and *Moksha* (liberation). The goal of liberating life can be achieved through perception and observations aided by a guru. The *Shrimad Bhagavad Gita* is often referred as the *Gita* is a narrative framework of dialogues between Pandava prince Arjuna and his mentor Lord Krishna, considered as the Avtar of Lord Vishnu. In *Gita*, *bhakti* (devotion) is characterized as the loving devotion, a longing, surrendered trust, and adoration of the divine guru Lord Krishna. Indian tradition of *Guru–Shishya* focuses upon formal and informal mentoring for the self-discovery and transformation.

India's diversity of culture can be seen in its people and their customs and habits. The role of guru in Indian tradition is that of spiritual counsellor, who helps mould values, shares more experiential knowledge, and acts as an inspirational person helping in the transformation of limitations to strengths. The shift from teacher guru to the mystic guru gained a great momentum during the seventh century AD with the rise of Bhakti Movement in India. The term 'guru' is also associated with being a mystic, who practices mysticism aiming for perfect union with the God.

In his book about neo-Hindu movements, Reender Kranenborg (2002, p. 50 quoted after Guru) distinguishes four types of gurus in India: 'The spiritual adviser', 'the enlightened master', the avatar or considered to be an incarnation of God, and a 'Guru' in the form of a book, that is Guru Granth Sahib in Sikh religion.

Vaishnavite traditions characterize gurus as persons who can show the path and can initiate one into *Sanyasa* order and spiritual education. The title guru (in Gurumukhi) is extremely important and fundamental to the Sikhism. The core beliefs of Sikhism are of belief in God and in the teachings of the Ten Gurus enshrined in Guru Granth Sahib, the holy book for Sikhs. Guru Nanak Dev Ji suggested about one god or *Akal* (timelessness), which permeates all life and can be seen with an inward eye or the heart of a human being.

The famous guru also suggested a lifestyle, doing actions such as *Kirat Karo*, *Nam Japo*, and *Wand Kay* meaning work diligently and honestly, mediate on the holy name (Wahe Guru), and share the fruits with others, respectively.

The enlightenment and empowerment spread through the messages of Guru had long-term implications for human welfare (*Seva*, selfless service), which is an integral part of Sikh religion and is widely practised for various philanthropic activities across the world. Sikhs always greet each other with the words 'Sat Sri Akal' which literally mean 'Truth is time less being'.

The tradition of *Guru–Shishya* and its exponents are followed by many in the Indian tradition whose influence was not only felt in the Indian society but also societies across the world. Even today, the traditions of yoga, classical music, and spiritual gurus have worldwide followers. In various Western countries, International Society for Krishna Consciousness, classical music gurus, and their traditions have large number of followers and practitioners. These teachings, preachings, and practices are relevant from the mental health point of view owing to its adherence to egoless attitude towards life and following the principle of service for humanity with universal orientation. The culture of *Guru–Shishya* tradition is so deep in Indian society that one particular day is celebrated as Guru Purnima paying respect to the teachers. In music field, the efficiency of a student can be judged on the basis of his/her training under a particular guru from a specific community of performers who have a distinctive musical style in common known as *Gharanas*. *Guru–Shishya* tradition always had a faith developed in its followers by the guru who can instil confidence and hope through regular interaction, discussing various conflicts and issues from a moralistic perspective.

Ayurveda

The word *veda* means knowledge. The evolution of the Indian tradition of healing and healthy life is derived from the four Vedas: *Rigveda*, *Samveda*, *Yajurveda*, and *Atharvaveda*. Ayurveda is one of the subsections of *Atharvaveda,* which deals with all forms of diseases and well-being techniques.

Charaka school of physicians (first century AD) and Sushruta school of surgeons (fourth century AD), known as *Charak Samhita* and *Sushruta Samhita*, became the basis of Ayurveda. Dridhabala in fourth century revised *Charak Samhita*. The texts of *Sushruta Samhita* were revised and suppressed by Nagarjuna in sixth century AD.

Ayurveda is divided into eight classes.

1) *Kaya-Chikitsa* (internal medicine)
2) *Baala Chikitsa* (treatment of children/pediatrics)
3) *Agada Tantra* (toxicology)
   Graha Chikitsa or Bhoot vidya (Psychiatry)
4) *Bhuta Vidya* (psychiatry)
   Urdhyaanga Chikitsa (treatment of eyes, nose throat, head related disease)
5) *Kaumara bhritya* (paediatrics).
   Shalyaroga chikitsa (surgery)
6) *Rasayana* (science of anti-aging)
   Damstra Chikitsa-Agad Tatra (toxicology)
7) *Vajikarana* (the science of fertility and aphrodisiac)
   Jara Chikitsa-Rasayana (geriatrics)
8) *Vrishta Chikitsa* or *Vajjikarna* (aphrodisiac therapy)

According to Charaka, Ayurveda denotes a combination of the body, sense organs, mind, and soul. Ayurveda suggests principle of *gunas* namely Sattwa, Rajas, and Tamas interweaving to create five elements that are space, air, fire, water, and earth, which gave birth to the entire creation.

Ayurveda suggests that everything in life is composed of the *panchamahabhutas: Akash* (space), *Vayu* (air), *Jal* (water), *Agni* (Fire), and *Prithvi* (Earth), constantly changing and interacting of which keeps the world going.

The uniqueness of Ayurveda is reflected in the intimate relationship between diet and mind.

Psychiatry in Ayurveda integrates mind, body, and soul.

Concept of Mind in Ayurveda

In the Ayurveda literature, physical mind is directly related to *Dhi* (intellect), *Dhruti* (processing information), and *Smruti* (memory). Three main constituents *vata*, *pitta*, and *kapha* are co-ordinating factors for good mental health.

Vata, *pitta*, and *kapha* are known as *Tridosha*. *Vata* governs the functioning of our nervous system, and an imbalance in it may cause psychological problems of anxiety, fears, or depression. In general, the endocrine/exocrine glandular activities are good pitta and musculoskeletal and anabolic system by Kapha. The seven *dhatus*, the basic tissues of the body, act as support when they are in a normal state. These are *rasa* (nutritive elements and product of gastrointestinal depression), *rakta* (blood), *mamsa* (muscle tissue), and *shukra* (reproductive elements). When normally disposed, the *dhatus* are in their 'prasada' state, that is fit for the body, and in a state of imbalance, they cause disease in the body.

The term *mala* means waste products, and *agni* corresponds to digestive elements involved in digestion and metabolism.

Ayurveda aims at maintaining equilibrium of *dosha*, *dhatu*, *mala*, and a health state of the *agni* (bio-fire).

The significance of *Trigunas* were emphasized by Charaka. Triguna is associated with mental orientation, and *vatta*, *pitta*, and *kapha* are related to anatomical and physiological characteristics. Sattva is considered the highest virtue of a person, which brings luminosity. Rajas is considered pleasure seeking, but any type of imbalance in it results into pain. *Tamas guna* is responsible for predominance of destructive actions and aggressions.

Rajas and *Tamas* are mainly responsible for psychological imbalance in a person.

According to Ayurveda, an excess of *Shaka* (sorrow), *Krodha* (anger), *Chinta* (unnecessary thinking), *Kama* (lust), *Lobha* (greed), *Moha* (delusion), *Irshya* (jealously), *Abhiamna* (pride), Mada (euphoric), and *Bhaya* (fear) are important negative emotions which can contribute to mental illness.

In Ayurveda, the therapy for mental illness is divided into three categories:

- *Daivavya prashraya*
- *Yukti-vya prashraya*
- *Sattva Vajaya chikitsa.*

Ayurveda also puts a great emphasis on yoga and lifestyle improvements. *Dinocharya* (daily routine) comprise an integral part of Ayurveda treatment with suggestions for rising early in the morning, choosing right foods, eating when hungry, and time for rest and play to be devoted for balanced growth.

Aachara Rasayana (self-conduct awareness) is a drugless treatment focusing on virtuous qualities to be maintained in life. One who speaks truth, abstains from alcohol and over indulgence, and maintains regular hygiene will have greater control over sense organs leading to physical, mental, and spiritual well-being.

Ayurveda is comprehensive approach of wellness which takes into account nutritional aspects, daily-routine aspects, behavioural aspects, breathing exercises, *pranayama*, and *niyam* (strict behavioural regime) which treat individuals from a holistic perspective and human being as a system not of isolated segment but of interrelated parts of our unified whole.

The fundamental principles of Ayurveda practice are derived from experience, which is ascertained by a fourfold examination, that is *atopadesha* (authoritative statement), *pratyaksha* (perception), *anumana* (inference), and *yukti* (*ranayama*) as stated in *Charak Samhita*.

In Ayurveda, substances of natural origin, many of which are used by pharmaceutical companies, including whole plants or their parts, animal parts, and minerals, are used as medicines either alone or in combination.

In case of imbalance of *dosha dhatu* and *mala*, the rational use of naturally available products aims to restore normality. It is no wonder that the majority of the household in India use Chyavanprash made from herbs (mainly) as a health improvement technique. It is worthwhile to maintain that Ayush Ministry suggested the use of Ayush-64 tablets for the treatment of mild COVID-19 patients.

It is a tradition of healing which is gaining its importance in Western countries, and the WHO also recognizes the oldest therapeutic system of Ayurveda being called traditional medicine or complementary and Alternative medicine are of the main objectives of the WHO traditional medicine strategy 2002–2005 to support countries to integrate traditional medicine into their own health system.

Yoga and Well-being

The chronology of texts describing Yoga is not very clear, but it is credited to *Upanishads* and *Yoga Sutra* of Patanjali (second century BCE). *Upanishads* are later *Vedic* era Sanskrit texts of religious teachings comprising the fundamentals of Hinduism. Yoga Sutra of Patanjali is a collection of Sanskrit sutras (aphorism) on the theory and practice of yoga (195 sutras according to Yvasa and 196 sutras according to some other scholars). The Yoga Sutra was compiled sometimes between 500 BC and 400 AD by the sage Patanjali. Later on with the efforts of Swami Vivekananda, the Theosophical Society gained Patanjali in twentieth century.

Patanjali divided his yoga sutras into four chapters (Sanskrit padas) containing 196 apharisms known as *Samadhi pada*, *Sadhna pada*, *Vibhuti pada*, and *Kaivalya pada*.

There are eight components of Yoga known as Ashtanga or the eight limbs: *Yama* (abstinences), *riyanma* (observances), asana (yoga postures), *pranayama* (breath, control), *pratyahara* (withdrawal of the senses), *dharna* (concentration), *dhyana* (meditation), and *samadhi* (absorption).

According to Patanjali, yoga is the control of mind (*chitta*) which is made of up of three components *manas*, *buddhi*, and *ahamkara*. Yoga philosophy suggests that mind is not the seer, but only an instrument of knowledge and real self or atman should be free from ego involvements. These are five kinds of thought wave: right knowledge, wrong knowledge, verbal delusion, sleep, and memory which can cause painful or not painful experiences.

In Patanjali's Yoga Sutra, practice and non-attachment are considered very useful qualities. Patanjali's Yoga Sutra suggests that concentration upon a single object may reach four different stages: examination, discrimination, joyful peace, and a single awareness of individuality. What is practised intensely can take the mind far, and it may reach the ultimate borders of undifferentiated matter.

During the stage of examination, mind gets perfectly concentrated upon one of the gross elements. The stage of discrimination is reached when mind penetrates the outer material and fastens upon *tanmatra*, the subtle essence within. The stage of 'joyful peace' is reached by concentrating upon the inner powers of perception. In the final stage of 'simple awareness of individuality', people concentrate upon the simplest ego-sense unmoved by any fear or desire. Knowing only that 'I' am other than this' or 'that' such stages are difficult to achieve but it is part of prakriti. The cosmic creation is considered as an evolution outward from undifferentiated into differentiated consciousness, that is from mind into matter.

Medication is a process considered as reverse of evolution, which begins at the surface and goes inward, till innermost reality is achieved. Faith recommended by Patanjali is flexible, provisional, and undogmatic, open to doubt and reason. Faith is not like a fixed entity, and it increases through personal experience and energy expands through practice. Patanjali reasons that the first teacher can only be God, and the word 'om; is used to express him.

From the psychology point of view, failure to concentrate results in distraction, causing grief, despondency, and breaking difficulties which can be overcome by the practices of concentration and meditation.

Yoga philosophy also emphasizes on cultivating happiness and having compassion for the unhappy and an attitude of forgiveness towards the wicked to secure calmness of mind.

Yoga also suggests the ability to develop extraordinary perception through superlative practice of concentration. *Samadhi* is of two types: *Nirvichara* (super-reflective) *Samadhi* is upon a subtle object which is unmixed with any other awareness, and *Suvichara Samadhi* (reflective) which is done upon a subtle object mixed with awareness of name, quality, and knowledge. In reaching *Nirvichara samadhi*, the mind becomes pure and transcendental.

From a yoga perspective, realization is the only goal of religion.

Nirvichara samadhi is a continuous consciousness of the unity of *Atman* and *Brahman* without any coverings for the *Atman*.

True austerity in Yoga is not a fantorical process of self-punishment but of quiet and same self-control in moderate ways.

The impediments on the way of enlightenment of a person are ignorance, egoism, and desire to cling to life, which are also highlighted in the *Gita*. People's tendency in contemporary times to seek security in the accumulation of possessions by violence is a misdirected notion of being happy.

In the philosophy of yoga, spiritual aspirants must not love things of this world too much, but we must not hate either as aversion creates a bondage of fear, and same applies to attachments. The law of Karma or action is expressively emphasized in yoga philosophy. According to Patanjali Yoga Sutra. the object of experience is composed of three *gunas* – the principle of illumination (*Sattwa*), activity (*Ragas*), and inertia (*Tamas*). These *gunas* pass through four states of gross, subtle, primal, and uninvolved. When the *guna* balance is in a state of equilibrium, their state is considered to be as unevolved. In case of disturbance in the guna balance, cosmic ego sense makes its presence felt; and when *gunas* enter into the combination which form the mind and the inner essence of things, this is considered as subtle state. At a point when *guna* reaches the external or physical manifestation, the state of *guna* is described as gross or defined.

The experience of consciousness reaches the highest of spiritual wisdom through different stages of perfect knowledge. The real source of all spiritual wisdom lies within a person, but, out of ignorance, people make long searches in churches and temples, where that is very near – in the Atman within them.

One of the eight limbs of yoga, *Yama*, indicates absenteeism from harming others. Another important limb *Niyama* prescribes purity of both physical and mental states.

When a person becomes steadfast in his abstention from inconsistence, it leads the way to acquire spiritual energy. The path of devotion towards God can be achieved through diverse ways. These are mentioned here.

Bhakti yoga: It is the path of loving, showing devotion to God.

Karma yoga: It is the selfless path of working with right means and god-dedicated action.

Jnana yoga: It is the path of intellectual discrimination and way of finding Brahman.

Raja Yoga: It is also called the yoga of meditation. It is also considered as vehicle of spiritual energy and wisdom.

The most famous asana is the lotus posture, and it is better to sit on the ground while doing asanas.

After mastering the posture, one can practice the control of *pranas* (*pranayama*) by stopping the motions of inhalation and exhalation. The inner light of spiritual wisdom can be achieved through the practice of *pranayama*.

Patanjali described that thought is a wave (*vritti*) in the mind and that practice of meditation (*dhyana*) is a unbroken flow of thought. Samadhi is a state of meditation in which the true nature of the object is not distorted by the perceiver.

The three constituents of concentration, meditation, and absorption in combination are called *Samyama*. However, 'seedless' samadhi (*nirvikalpa*) demands more spiritual energy. It is a stage when all mental distractions disappear, and the mind becomes single-focused. The goal of mental health experts is to overcome distractions through use of psychotherapy. *Samayama* is the way to acquire delightful knowledge about the past, present, and future.

Yoga from a psychological perspective is important, and it is more relevant from a medical point of view. Yoga practices have the ability to lower cortical levels which can boost our immune system. Excessive cortisol secretion has been linked with major depression, high blood pressure, and insulin resistance.

Asana and *pranayama* are empirically known sources to improve immune functioning, and meditation has a strong scientific support in this area.

Relaxation through yoga exercises also helps in muscular and nervous system relaxation.

Scientific evidences also support the contention that specific hearth rhythms generate brain-wave patterns which can raise the temperature of hands.

When one regularly keeps heart rate in aerobic ranges, one can lower the risk of heart attack and can relieve depression. Yoga activities were frequently done during the times of pandemic to improve oxygen levels in the body.

The patients of blood pressure get relieved from their problems by the use of Savasana technique of yoga.

Hatha yoga, through holding static physical postures (asanas), uses stretching and improves muscular strength and flexibility so that it is likely to be beneficial for some musculoskeletal problems.

Yoga activities affect every cell of the body through better neurotransmitter communication and increase resistance against stress. Yoga as a method of exercise is widely performed in schools, colleges, and other sections of the population in majority of the countries of the world. The International Yoga Day is celebrated annually on 21 June since 2015 following its inception in the United Nations General Assembly in 2014.

Yoga can induce harmony in mind, body and soul, and this has proved to be a very powerful technique for mental health improvement. It has an immense potential to help in sustaining wellness and act as a preventive as well as curative technique to empower an individual's physical and mental health.

Psychology researchers need to play an important role to increase the awareness of different forms of yoga and also try to mitigate the myths and stereotypes preventing its use by the masses. Yoga as a way life comprising mental, physical, and spiritual integration to achieve sustainable wellness can be a game-changer in wellness paradigms, which can be very useful for working and old population.

Music and Well-being

The psychologist of music seeks the neatest and most economical manner of describing music's structure in a way that most closely resembles processes by which music is created, reproduced and understood (Sloboda, 1985, p. 11).

In the past, some Greek theorists and subsequently Pythagoras suggested some correspondence between physical facts (the vibration frequency) and facts of sensation (pitch).

Fechner in addition is said to have established psycho-physics and its experimental methods (1906) and also created the field what is today known as experimental aesthetics (1876). Helmholtz (1877/1995) examined the generalizable psycho-acoustic aspects of musical sounds rather than individual taste.

The psychology of music as a field studies several domains such as emotional and aesthetic response to music, role of music in healing mental illness, and other aspects related to it. Music psychology shares interdisciplinary relations with the fields of psycholinguistics and ethnomusicology. Psycholinguistics deal with relations between language and music and the role of culture in the acquisition of such skills.

Movement as Expressive Gesture

Music performer's movement encompass, sound and non-sound producing movements related to expressive goals. The term 'expressive gestures' refers both to acoustic cues that distinguish one performance of the same music from another and motion cue of musicians' bodies and instruments that often highlight important aspects of performance (Palmer, 1997; Wanderley, 2002). For example visual cues such as the head and upper torso movements of performing points can be as effective as auditory cues in conveying the pianists' intended expressivity to views (Davidson, 1995). A strong positive correlation has been found with the movements and acoustic features of instrumental artists' expressive performance.

Delande (1988) classified the possible gestures of a musician into three basic categories: effective gestures, figurative gestures, and accompanying gestures. Accompanying or ancillary gestures are visible movements not directly related to sound production but having the capability to influence perceivers' judgements.

Some musicians also examine body movements that synchronize with periodicities present in music. It is assumed on the basis of researches that the motion of individual performers can enhance sensory information to guide the timing and dynamics of performance, having impact on viewers' judgements.

Ensemble performance and sensory impact

Majority of issues relating to psychology of music focus more on individual aspects of performance. The group performance in music occurs between musicians in groups, from duets to large orchestral ensembles. Ensemble performance requires individual to adapt to sensorimotor integration in the group situation. Seminal studies of solo and choral singing have documented changes in articulation, phonation, and overall sound level when singers perform together in ensembles (Rossing et al., 1986). The ability and skills of music artists in producing synchronicity may decide its impact on viewers. Temporal coordination plays a dominant part in the performance of ensembles. The audience performance anxiety of the artists is also influenced by the social factor of non-vital cues from the audience.

Music Performance

Music performances provide diverse resources for the study of cognitive and motor skills. Psychological studies aim to study music performance factors, choices the performers make, and the relationship between performance and perception.

Each performer has his or her skill and intention to convey musical composition to their viewers or listeners. A crucial aspect of music presentation involves conveying the emotional contact of the music.

A great degree of importance and attention is required to strike a balance of relationships among melodic, harmonic, and diatonic elements. Knowledge of diatonic and harmonic structure influences the performance of the musicians.

Another standard yardstick overcoming the individual interpretations is style-specific syntactic properties of meter providing temporal framework in the performance. Schenker's (1969) music theory views the melodic and harmonic organization of a musical piece as a series of progressively more complex elaboration of a simple foundation, the background from which the surface level is generated one of the first types of musical structure for which systematic pattern of performance expression were documented is the duration patterns that form characteristic rhythms perceptual experiments suggest that listeners can apprehend the music theoretic perditions of melodic expectancies (Cuddy & Luney, 1995; Krumhansl, 1995) and tension-relaxation (Krumhansl, 1996) from just the categorical score information presented in computer generated (expressionless) performances.

Tempo and Temporal Structure

Tempo refers to the pace of music or the rate at which musical events unfold over time (McAuley, 2010). The tempo is strongly associated with beat rate (i.e. beats per minute, bpm), and other factors like event density, register, and loudness also influence its perception.

Memory for tempo and rhythm is considered to be robust and objective.

Music is enjoyed in a situation when the body movements lock in and synchronize with music. The perception of accents also forms a crucial part through which certain events are perceived to be more salient than others.

MRI (Magnetic Resonance Imaging) and EEG (Elctroencephalogram) studies have identified brain areas such as basal ganglia as well as auditory cortex as the key components that can sense the feeling of entertainment. The superiority of musicians to deconstruct and organize a rhythm's temporal structure may relate to the greater involvement of the prefrontal cortex in mediating working memory and may possibly involve the documented leftward shift as musical expertise increases (Bhattacharya & Petsche, 2005; Kuchenbuch et al., 2012).

Groove is defined as 'the urge to move in the response to music, combined with the positive affect associated with the coupling of sensory and motor processes remote engaging with music' (Janata et al., 2012, p. 54). Groove becomes a basis for getting a pleasurable experience from certain musical rhythms, compelling us to move.

Synesthesia, is vivid precepts arise in one modality due to stimulation in another modality (Talsama et al., 2009).

Music involves a superior quality reception and perception of melodic impact having a positive influence on the listeners. Greater level of attention and meaningful involvement with the music can head to flow experiences to its practitioners and the listeners. Desirable sound of music has a wide range of psychological implications with positive impact on mood, enhanced effect, and other healing effects. The impact of music also relates to learning, improving memory, perception, and attention, which are useful for mental health. The motivational level and endurance capacities are also improved with music therapy methods. Moreover, studies have shown that music with the combination of exercise can alleviate symptoms of stress. Music enhances brain function in reading, reasoning, and memorizing in human (Miendiarzewska & Trost, 2014). Kuhn (2002) demonstrated that a particular type of music can create a positive and profound emotional experience, which leads to the secretion of immune-boosting hormones resulting in reduction in factors related to many illnesses. Several music intervention programmes are found to the extremely useful to overcome depression and stress.

Critical Evaluation

The relationship between spirituality and mental health well-being is relatively less researched and less practised for therapeutic purposes. The pre-dominance of DSM model of treatment focuses mostly on individual centric problems whereas the real focus should integrate social, cultural, and other subjective dimensions of the problem. The current system of ICD and DSM classification do a lot in labelling persons ignoring the intuition, creativity, and spirituality aspects. Besides that, many commentators accuse DSM of what they call 'hyponarrativity', a term coined by psychiatrist John Z. Sadler, meaning that signs and symptoms of a mental disorder can be assessed empirically and independently of the subjective experiences of the patient, or the circumstances of his life, and of the personal meaning the patient ascribes to them as well as to his symptoms. The tendency of this model eliminating subjective experiences and interpersonal contact in order to reach a scientific analysis of mental disorders is not a holistic approach.

Diagnostic criteria used by clinicians are certainly useful in a large variety of situations, but so many aspects of reality like altered states of consciousness and dimensions of spiritual experience are not given due importance. It was proved that the consensual neo-Kraeplinian descriptions of syndromes not only failed to serve as an adequate basis for etiological research, but, to a great extent, they also became unintended 'epistemic prison' for clinical and translational researchers (*Annual Rev. Clin Psychology*, 2016 , 12: 435–463).

The aspects of bliss, wisdom, community traditions and beliefs, religious faiths, and coping abilities are excluded in the objective diagnostic criteria. The huge role of statistics and big data approach to combine the genotype–phenotype factors at times ignores subjective experience.

The debates have emerged for alternative model based upon multitudes of distinct environmental, chromosomal, and spiritual aspects, It is also desirable to look into the developments in virtual activities and their implications on human behaviour in the contemporary circumstances. Culture and belief systems of indigenous communities should be taken into account to extend diverse dimensions of the diagnostic criteria.

One of the dominant claims of evolutionary psychology regarding brain as a collection of cognitive adaptations and idea of multimodular mind does not find adequate space in this existing model of DSM/ICD classification. There is considerable need for deconstructing latent variables' role to determine the spectrum of psycho-pathology. Alternative approaches comprising diverse cultural and spiritual practices existing in diverse indigenous locations should be given their due importance.

The tendency of pharmaceuticalization are problems always amenable to pharmaceutical intervention is disquieting. Attending to plurality of perspective faith and healing can certainly add to our understanding of psychopathology. Sociological and spiritual analysis can help in mapping several new dimensions related to mental health ecology. It is not being suggested to question the capability of diagnostic methods, but adding more dimensions will make its understanding better and realistic.

The concepts like mindfulness, yoga meditation, and Ayurveda practices can transform our understanding to a deeper level with their implications for well-being. The process of ambivalence in inclusion or exclusion of disorders from the manual is often influenced by extraneous factors, and these changes are influenced by the social climate of opinion raised and highlighted by advocacy groups.

Diagnostic labels are powerful and may hurt people, and influencing dimensions need to be explored and examined to reach an appropriate understanding of this issue.

Summary

The goal of spirituality is to transcend I-centred consciousness and eliminate that which separates one from cosmic existence. The notion of liberation is not found in forceful acts designed to create a better world, but it can be achieved through decentring of individualistic concerns for the benefit of the society as a whole. Endless bliss and equanimity are the highest goals of a wise man. In order to cultivate an ethical and spiritual orientation, good company (*satsanga*), making one's conduct virtuous (*sadachara*), and heeding the teachers (guru) are essential components. Spirituality focuses more upon human efforts and creativity and is a result of one's own consciousness.

A growing evidence of research has found that spirituality enhances mental health, and well-being spirituality has several dimensions of religiosity, mystic experiences, transcendence, sacrifice, and other methods; level of transcendence called intrapersonal is known as an individual's capacity to know and nourish one's own self also known as inner strength. The other type of transcendence is one's connectedness that one has with God, also considered as higher powers of consciousness.

All spiritual experiences provide a meaning in life as they are considered to enable motivation and empowerment, providing a ground for robust self-identity. The relationship and connectedness to supreme can be achieved by one's devotion of highest value, and this can be someone's work or any other activity such as social service. However, Indian perspective of spirituality sees it as being interconnected on the same continuum, and elevated understanding self can lead to transcendence. Mystical experiences are considered to be important constituents of spiritual experiences leading to higher states of motivation and flow experiences. Two tendencies of saintliness have the natural capability for inculcation of charity, purity, self-sacrifice, and self-surrender contributing to healthier mental states. It has been found through empirical evidences that people having religious and mystical orientation have high levels of subjective well-being. Religious and spiritual orientations are similar in their striving to the transcendent, and they also support altruistic activities. However, there are some differences in terms of emphasis on ritual aspects in case of religion which may not be present in spiritual aspects. Spirituality may help a person to cope with misery through hope, faith, and trust.

Spirituality helps in coping through alternations in the sense of getting meaning in life. These several characteristic traits found to the dominant in the religious and spiritual persons.

Gratitude as a trait is accorded greater importance. Regular expressions of gratitude lead to increased feelings of happiness and greater life satisfaction. People involved in religious and spiritual activities often direct their activities for the benefit of others. Gratitude helps people feel more positive emotions, and it helps in developing ability to handle adversity. People who regularly express gratitude for the positive things are considered to be happier, and this can lead to lower levels of stress and depression. Gratitude as a social emotion also helps in building effective interpersonal relationships. The construct of hope plays a crucial role in the healthy mental process. Hope is considered to be positive in planning to meet goals. Hopeful individuals pose positive sense of thinking, leading to optimism and satisfaction. An individual's ability to bounce back in adversity is positively affected with high hopes. Possessing hope and resilience positively affects an individual's mood and functioning.

A sense of hope is also associated with a reduced risk of stress and fewer sleep problems. Trait hope involves the belief that one can produce 'routes to desired goals' (Snyder & Snyder, 2008). Hope is also considered as a positive indicator of quality adjustments.

The process of recovery for people suffering from different problems depends a lot on people themselves that they desire to get better. The journey of recovery is an ongoing, personal process which aims to allow a person to have satisfied life despite adversities posed by their conditions.

Indian perspective of the law of Karma refers to good activities leading to good consequences striving for positivity and hope. Healing is achieved through balance between inner and outer realities, and seeking harmony is the central pillar of self-realization. Rao highlights Vivekanand's view on hope saying 'we must love others because others are no other than ourselves'. Thus love becomes the cardinal virtue, which along with hope and optimism guides our conduct. Altruism is the opposite of selfishness: it involves detachment as opposed to attachment (Aasakti) which is source of all misery. Hope is the driving, force. Infinite hope infinite aspiration (Vivekananda Vol. 3, p. 443; Rao, 2014, p. 101).

Vivekananda stated that people with religious and spiritual orientations have high hopes owing to faith in beliefs of compassion, altruism, and generativity. The activities of prayers and meditation are good predictors of perceived hope.

Forgiveness is also considered to be a moral virtue to generate positive emotional feelings within a person. Forgiveness can help a person release deep feelings of resentment and overcome negative thoughts.

Genuine forgiveness requires compassion, benevolence, and love for the offender with the relinquishment of the tendency to take revenge. Religiosity and spirituality emphasize the social–moral mechanisms for forgiveness. Good relational qualities and good mental health can be sustained through the qualities of forgiveness. The interventions on forgiveness measures also contribute to the hope and optimism.

Indian traditions of spirituality like Ayurveda, yoga, music, and *Guru–Shishya* tradition can be meaningful contributors to mental health and well-being. There is a need to complement the existing scientific models of diagnosis and prognosis by exploring alternative approaches to mental health and well-being. These Indian approaches are based upon meaningful principles of harmony between mind, body, and soul and with a lot of emphasis on inner balances and self-reliance. It does not categorize feelings on good/bad dichotomies; instead, it tends to treat them in continuum. It they more upon the exploration of qualities within a person and is less dependent on external persons to care about the problems. Healthy mind is abode of healthy body, which results in healthy behaviour. It focuses upon a strict discipline of food, good conduct, sacrifice, self-control, and altered states of consciousness to achieve a harmonious growth in life.

Think Box

What role can spirituality play in maintaining a healthy state of mind and body? In this context, discuss the Indian perspective and its contribution.

Key Points:

- Spirituality is referred to contrast with materialistic ways of being and contact with spirits and psychological phenomenon of transcendence.
- The existential approach suggests that the dialectic between nature and freedom is repeated in human situations.
- The experience of consciousness is personal to each person, and it is always different from that of others.
- Mystical experiences vary in intensity and generally involve an experience of transcendence beyond normal categories.
- Bereavement or the loss of loved ones can be less painful for the spiritually mature persons.
- Gratitude is a commonly experienced emotion also conceptualized as an attitude, a moral virtue, a personality trait, and a coping response.
- As a social emotion, expressions of gratitude and appreciation are contributors to long-term interpersonal relationships.
- Depression and negative life events are less intense for those who are hopeful.
- One who unconditionally forgives also is happy because the anger on the forgiven is exterminated.
- India's diversity of culture can be seen in its people and their customs and habits.

Key Terms:

Mysticism, Secular, Spirituality, Religion, Rational, Ineffability, *Guru–Shishya* tradition, Yoga music, Forgiveness, Well-being

References

Allport, G. W. (1966). The religious context of prejudice. *Journal for the Scientific study of Religion*, *5*, 447–457.

Allport, G. W., & Ross, J. M. (1967). Personal. Religious orientation and prejudice. *Journal of Personality and Social Psychology, 5*, 432–443.

Batson, C. D., & Schoenrade, P. A. (1991). Measuring religious quest: Validity concerns. *Journal for the Scientific Study of Religion, 30*, 416–429.

Batson, C. D., Schonerade, P. A., & Ventis, W. L. (1993). *Religion and the individual: A social-psychological perspective*. Oxford University Press.

Benson, C. K. (1992). Forgiveness and the psychotherapeutic process. *Journal of Psychology and Christianity, 11*, 76–81.

Bhattacharya, J., & Petsche, H. (2005). Phase synchrony analysis of EEG during music perception reveals changes in functional connectivity due to musical expertise. *Signal Process, 85*(11), 21, 61–77.

Cuddy, L. L., & Luney, C. A. (1995). Expectancies generated by melodic intervals: Perceptual judgements of melodic continuity percept. *Psychophysics, 57*, 451–462.

D'Aquili, E. G., & Newberg, A. B. (2000). The neuropsychology of aesthetic, spiritual, and mystical states. *Zygon, 35*, 39–51.

Davidson, J. W. (1995). What does the visual information contained in music performances after the observer: Some preliminary thoughts. In R. Steinberg (Ed.), *Music and the mind machine* (pp. 105–114). Springer.

Delande, F. (1988). La gestique de Gould. In G. Guertain (Ed.), *Glenn Gould puriel* (pp. 85–111). Louise, Courteau Editrice.

Edwards, J. (2004). *The religious affections*. Banner of Truth Trust.

Enright, R. D., Freedman, S., & Rique, J. (1998). The psychology of interpersonal forgiveness. In R. D. Enright & J. North (Eds.), *Exploring forgiveness* (pp. 46–62). University of Wisconsin Press.

Erikson, F. (1966). Ontogeny of ritualization. In R. Lowenstein, L. Newman, M. Schur, & A. Solnit (Eds.), *Psychoanalysis – A general psychology: Essays in honor of Heinz Hartmann* (pp. 601–621). International University Press.

Fechner, G. T. (1876). *Vorschule der Aesthetik [Propaedeutics of aesthetics]*. Breitkopf & Härtel.

Fechner, G. T. (1906). *On life after death, from the German of Gustav Theodor Fechner [Das Büchlein vom Leben nach dem Tode]* (H. Wernekke, Ed. and Trans.; pp. 7–134). Open Court Publishing Co.

Ferguson, F. (2001). Personality and coping traits: A joint factor analysis. *British Journal of Health Psychology, 6*, 311–395.

Folkman, S., & Lazarus, R. S. (1985). If it changes it must be a process: Study of emotion and Coping during three stages of a college examination. *Journal of Personality and Social Psychology, 48*, 150–170.

Fowler, J. W. (1996). *Faithful change: The personal and public challenges of postmodern life*. Abingdon.

Fowler, J. W., & Dell, M. L. (2004). Stages of faith and identity: Birth to teens. *Child and Adolescent Psychiatric Clinics of North America, 13*(1), 17–33.

Girad, R. (1977). *Violence and the sacred* (P. Gregory, Trans). John Hopkins University Press.

Harrington, T. A., & Blankenship, V. (2002). Rumination thoughts and their relation to depression and anxiety. *Journal of Applied Social Psychology, 32*, 465–485.

Helmholtz, H. (1877/1995). *On thought in medicine* (E. Atkinson, Trans.). Longmans.

Hood, R. W. Jr. (2001). *Dimensions of mystical experiences; Empirical studies and psychological links*. Rodopi.

Hope, D. (1987). The healing paradox of forgiveness. *Psychotherapy, 24*, 240–244.

James, W. (1961). *The varieties of religious experience* (pp. 299–300). Collier. (Original work published 1902).

Janata, P., Tomic, S. T., & Haberman, J. (2012). Sensorimotor coupling in music and the psychology of the groove. *Journal of Experimental Psychology: General, 141*(1), 54–75.

Jeringon, H. L. (2001). Spirituality in older adults: A cross-cultural and interfaith perspective. *Pastoral Psychology, 49*, 413–437.

Krumhansl, G. L. (1995). Music psychology and music theory: Problems and prospects. *Music Theory Spectrum, 17*, 53–80.

Krumhansl, G. L. (1996). A perceptual analysis of Morat, piano sonata, K.282 segmentation tension and musical ideas. *Music Perception, 13*, 401–432.

Kuchenbuch, A., Paraskevopoulos, E., Herholz, S. C., & Pantev, C. (2012). Electromagnetic correlates of musical expertise in processing of tone patterns. *PLoS ONE, 7*(1), e30171.

Kuhn, D. (2002). The effects of active and passive participation in musical activity on the immune system as measured by salivary immunoglobulin A (SlgA). *Journal of Music Therapy, 39*(1), 30–39.

Maslow, A. H. (1999). *Toward a psychology of being* (3rd ed., p. 98). John Wiley & Sons.

May, G. (2004). *The dark night of the soul: A psychiatrist explores the connection between darkness and spiritual growth*. Harper San Francisco.

McAuley, J. D. (2010). Tempo & rhythm. In M. R. Jones (Ed.), *Music perception* (pp. 165–199). Springer. Music & Mental Health.

McCullough, M. E., & Worthington, E. L. Jr. (1994). Encouraging Clients to forgive people who have hurt them. Review, critique and research prospectus. *Journal of Psychology and Theology, 22*, 3–20.

Miendlarzewska, E. A., & Trost, W. J. (2014). How musical training affects cognitive development: Rhythm, reward and other modulating variables. *Frontiers in Neuroscience, 142*(2), 1–18.

Neibuhr, R. (1966a). *The nature and destiny of man: A Christian interpretation: Volume 7. Human nature*. Westminster John Knox Press (Original work published 1948).

Neibuhr, R. (1966b). *The nature and destiny of man: A Christian interpretation: Volume II. Human destiny*. Westminster John, Knox Press (Original York Published 1943).

Otto, R., & Otto, d. (1950). *The idea of holy* (2nd ed.). (J. Harvey, Trans.). Oxford University Press (Original work published 1923).

Palmer, C. (1997). Music performance. *Annual Review of Psychology, 48*, 115–138.

Pargament, K. I. (1990). God help me. Toward a theoretical framework of coping for the Psychology of religion. *Research in the Social Scientific Study of Religion, 2*, 195–224.

Pargament, K. I. (1997). *The Psychology of religion and coping. Theory, research and practice* (New ed.). Guilford.

Rao, K. R. (2014). Positive psychology and Indian psychology in need of mutual reinforcement, *Psychological Studies, 59*(2), 94–102.

Reiss, S., & Havercamp, S. M. (1998). Toward a comprehensive assessment of fundamental motivation: Factor structure of the Reiss profiles. *Psychological Assessment, 10*(2), 97–106.

Roehlkepartain, E. (2004). The co-construction of spiritual meaning in parent-child communication. In D. Ratcliff (Ed.), *Children's spirituality: Christian perspectives, research and applications* (pp. 182–200). Cascade.

Rossing, T. D., Sundberg, J., & Transtran, S. (1986). Acoustic comparisons of Soparano Solo and chair singing. *Journal of Acoustic Society of America, 79*, 1975–1981.

Sarkar, R. (2011). *The bird image, in Savitri: Sradha – A quarterly devoted to an exposition of the teachings of the Mother and Sri Aurobindo* (Vol. 2, No. 4, Special Issue on Saviri, Part-II, pp. 73–97). Sri Aurobindo (Centre for Research in Social Sciences).

Schaefer, C. A., & Gorsuch, R. L. (1992). Dimensionality of religion: Belief and motivation as predictors of behavior. *Journal of Psychology and Christianity, 11*(3), 244–254.

Schenker, H. (1969). *Graphic music analysis*. Dover.

Sloboda, J. (1985). *The music mind: The cognitive psychology of music*. Clarendon Press.

Snyder, L. G., & Snyder, M. J. (2008). Teaching critical thinking and problem solving skills. *Delta Pi Epsilon Journal, 50*, 90–99.

Talsama, D., Senkowski, D., & Woldorff, M. G. (2009). Intermodal attention affects the processing of the temporal alignment of audiovisual stimuli. *Experimental Brain Research, 198*(2–3), 313–328.

Temoshok, L. R., & Chandra, P. S. (2000). The meaning of forgiveness is a specific situational and cultural context. In M. E. McCullough, K. T. Paragament, & C. E. Theresen (Eds.), *Forgiveness; Theory, research practice* (pp. 45–64). Guilford Press.

Vergote, A. (2003). Playing between psychology and mysticism. In J. Belzen & A. Geels (Eds.), *Mysticism: A variety of psychological perspectives* (pp. 81–107). Rodopi.

Vivekananda, S. (2015). *The complete works of Sami Vivekananda*. Manonmani Publishers.

Wanderley, M. M. (2002). Quantitative analysis of non-obvious performer gestures. In I. Wachsmuth & T. Sowa (Eds.), *Gesture and Sign Languages in human computer interaction* (pp. 241–252). Springer Verlag.

Winnicott, D. W. (1975). *Through paediatrics to psycho-analysis: Collected papers*. Brunner/Mazel.

Winnicott, D. W. (1990). *The maturational process and the facilitating environment* (pp. 100–101). Karnac Books.

Worthington, E. L. Jr., Bertry, J. W., & Parrott, L. III (2001). Unforgiveness, forgiveness, religion and health. In T. G. Plante & A. C. Sherman (Eds.), *Faith and health psychological perspectives* (pp. 107–138). Guilford Press.

Worthington, E. L., Jr., & Wade, N. G. (1999). The psychology of unforgiveness and forgiveness and implications for clinical practice. *Journal of Social and Clinical Psychology, 18*(4), 385–418.

7 Suffering and Healing

Learning Objectives

After reading this chapter, you will be able to understand:

- The concepts of suffering and healing
- Eastern and Western perspective
- Buddhism perspective
- The *Bhagavad Gita* perspective
- Interdisciplinary perspective

Introduction

A comprehensive definition of suffering according to Cassell (2004) is 'the state of severe distress associated with events that threaten the intactness of person' (p. 32). Healing to Cassell is restoring the intactness by reassembling parts or aspects of a person in a new manner. Cultural norms and socio-historical contextual experiences are essential to understand the concepts of suffering and healing.

Suffering and healing are not limited to physiological symptoms, and they are also influenced a lot by moral and spiritual meanings. Suffering can also occur when people have lost their loved ones, events, objects, or positions in life. People are subject to this kind of suffering because of the web of relationship with self and others. Healing on the other hand is a bouncing back ability to recover from distressing circumstances.

How culture shapes suffering becomes clear from Lewis-Fernández and Kleinman's (1994) definition of culture 'as value commitments and moral orientations more akin to faith that are embodied in, experienced by individuals as what is at stake in specific local setting' (p. 68). People also suffer when he/she is unable to meet the social–moral expectations of the society members and family members.

From a spiritual perspective, suffering is the necessary condition for spiritual growth. The insightful moments and meaning that come through sacrifice of suffering can lead to self-transcendence. Christ's suffering on the cross

DOI: 10.4324/9781003350651-7

became a paradigm case for positive suffering. Godly incarnations and pious souls suffered to send mankind the message of stop doing evil. Lord Rama suffered to set an ideal to humanity. Dispassionate follower of *Dharma* and Karma cycle is a bondage that keeps one trapped in the illusions of pleasure and pain. But the moment one overcomes this binary of attachments to pain and pleasures, they are detached from the lust of desires and they move towards liberation whose ultimate aim is *Moksha*.

The first noble truth of Buddhism focuses upon the fact that 'life is suffering'. The *Bhagavad Gita* very succinctly and clearly explains that the root cause of human suffering is attachment. From a social constructionist approach, suffering and healing arise in socio-moral contexts of human existence. Psychological reality of a person can't be independent of the observer, and reality is constructed through situated exchanges between people. Suffering and healing are processes that are constituted through the interactions between healers and sufferers. The meaning of suffering is different for different people varying along socio-cultural dimensions, and it is inherently subjective, local, and pluralistic in nature.

Gergen (1994) argues that the attempts of the mental health professionals to reduce the dehumanization biomedicine causes the afflicted persons to 'remain lodged, for the most part, in the realist view of mental events and belief that these can be no objectively current accounts of the interior world' (p. 162). The person-centred dogma derived from social institution medicine confines sickness or suffering to biological symptoms. Gergen (1994) contends that the use of language to describe mental states like 'attitude', 'anxiety', or 'feelings' in a referential manner (presuming that language represents mental states existing 'out their' within the individual independent of language) can mislead us towards what he called fallacy of misplaced concreteness. The attitude of medicalization of diagnostic labels experience a feeling of community erosion in the sets of life lived before being diagnosed and after being diagnosed.

The element of fear and stereotypes from movies and television impact a well-managed person suddenly diagnosed with some disorders. Charmaz (2002) talked about silenced suffering and argued

> ill people intentionally remain silent when they believe that (a) other people cannot comprehend their situations (b) their views would hurt a significant person (c) voicing them would prove too costly and or (d) no one wants to hear the story.
>
> (p. 309)

Culturally authorized meanings and interpretation also play a crucial role in suffering and healing: compassion and empathy are the methods through which a caregiver can understand the suffering of a client.

Klienman (1998) has recommended the way of mini-ethnography and a brief life history as methods that may gain insights into illness experiences.

The role of understanding subjective experiences of suffering is highlighted by Cassell (2004) as he asserts, 'with a few exceptions, the worldview knowledge and disciplines trying to gain entrance to medicine and purity in the curriculum are based on the subjective' (p. xiv). Marsella (1998) emphasizes that qualitative research approaches are suited to the study of subjective experiences as he mentions, 'qualitative research openly acknowledges the interpretive influence of the researcher in arriving at conclusion, in doing so it legitimizes and endorses subjective research approaches' (p. 1287).

Adequate compassion and an interdisciplinary approach to understand the local should be accorded adequate attention while trying to explore suffering and healing. Social suffering is experienced by the people who encounter conflicts and discrimination due to socio-cultural deprivations. David Morris (1991, 1998) argues about cultural account of suffering and maintains that people's experiences of suffering are always relative to the particular cultural narratives through which they relate to exigencies of self and others. From a social point of view, suffering is not a private act, rather it is a socially and culturally co-constructed phenomenon.

One of the most famous contributions in the field of social suffering is that of Pierre Bourdieu's. The weight of the world social suffering in contemporary society (1999).

Bourdieu has argued about the painful part of lived experiences of social domination and exclusion and its psychic implications for negative social experiences. Another pioneer work done in this field is by Veena Das and Arthur Klienman who have described the ways in which societies try to cope with suffering they produce and define legitimate discursive and practical reactions to this suffering.

Collective suffering of the people is labelled as social pathology, and its solutions are social and political in nature.

Social suffering can't be dealt with philosophical orientation, and its solutions need to be found in political public sphere.

For example the discrimination on the basis of caste in India causes a huge social suffering, and its solutions can be found in political spheres of governance. On the normative side, it seems reasonable to suggest that structurally produced suffering of social order and social context acts as a serious obstacle in the self-potential realization by discriminated categories of people.

Feelings of insecurity pervade among the members of low-income underclass and street children. With the onset of market economy and popularizational public sector institutions, the collective situation of safety, health, and education has deteriorated for the marginals sections of the society. Far from integrating the social underclass into the mainstream, they are reconverted into instruments of surveillance and policing of a surplus population that must be warehoused in the ghetto of urban. Public authority of slums turns into a machine against the poor by isolating these marginal sections into stigmatized social space of slums.

Poverty and insecurity create a vicious cycle of suffering. Poverty-related discrimination and mental health problems are shaped by wide-ranging inequalities of social, economic, and physical environment in which people live, The experience of homelessness and economic hardship induces a complex trauma affecting such people's emotional abilities and relationships.

Stigma and discrimination affect people being internalized by them, which have silencing effects on them, preventing and seeking support.

There are cumulative impacts of unemployment, material conditions, parental attitude, and various other factors which result in inequitable mental health outcomes.

Adverse childhood experiences of the poor children act as a contributor in the disruption of child's psychological, health, and personality development.

The children who spend their early childhood in streets, without homes, or in ghetto of slums are impacted by a lack of attachment and exposure to neglect and physical and psychological abuse which may result in severe behavioural problems. Neglectful parenting and maltreatment are common experiences faced by children born in poverty, and these cumulative stressors cause suffering resulting into mental health problems. Psycho-social conditions of inequalities impact health conditions through the perception of social exclusion and loneliness. Stigma caused by poverty acts as contributor to low self-esteem, social isolation, and delayed help seeking. People with low socio-economic status experiencing hunger and debt are more likely to suffer from mental disorders in comparison to affluent persons with high economic status.

The relationship between mental ill health and poverty is also cyclical in nature. Poverty increases the risk of mental disorders, and having a mental disorder increases the likelihood of descending into poverty.

Violence against women is another significant cause of suffering amongst Indian women though it is a global problem as well.

Violence against women by their partners and sexual violence can negatively affect women's physical and mental health.

The United Nations defines violence against women as

> [A]ny act of gender based violence that results in, or is likely to result in physical, sexual or mental harm or suffering to women, including threats of such acts, coercion or arbitrary deprivation of liberty, whether occurring in public or private life.
>
> (United Nations, 1993)

Violence against women and the girl child are important contributors to health problems.

Long exposure to violence is strongly associated with high risk of depression, anxiety and post-traumatic stress disorders. The data collected from police sources present a picture of reported cases of crime against women, and the number of unreported cases of violence against women is extremely high in number. The suffering related to violence against women has direct and indirect implications for mental health issues.

Caste Discrimination and Suffering

The untouchables in India are at the bottom of caste hierarchy in terms of poverty index, unemployment, and housing and health aspects.

Caste is a complex social and psychological construct in which concepts of social hierarchy feature prominently during the interactions between high and low castes. Gorringe and Rafanell (2007) highlighted three dimensions of caste: 1) social hierarchy, in which status is privileged over economic and political power; 2) endogamous separation, in which inter-marriage between other castes is discouraged and forbidden; and 3) an interdependent division of labour.

Caste functions as an important social unit in the villages of India governing personal and social relationships leading to prejudice and caste-based atrocities.

Social identity approaches indicate that individuals may come to regard themselves as interchangeable exemplars of their social groups by viewing themselves and others primarily in terms of their caste group memberships (Turner et al., 1987).

Caste identity also influences individuals' self-concept, and it has implications to a self-esteem and psychological coherence.

The social prejudice against lower-caste people is still prevalent in rural parts of the country. The prejudice-related activities range from verbal abuse to physical violence resulting in a state of psycho-social suffering for the members of underprivileged castes.

Although untouchability is illegal under the constitution of India, but there are several cases of physical violence still reported from various parts of the country to enforce illegal rules. There are three dimensions of untouchability: exclusion from public spaces and public water sources and humiliation and exploitation by the high castes (e.g. Deshpande, 2011). Under the caste system, which still prevails in rural India, preeminence is assigned to birth rather than competition (Beteille, 2011).

The social discrimination based on caste identity has human development implications on education and health. Caste mediated by gender and class, among other things, affects millions of people, and yet we know little about the mechanisms or experiences of social suffering involved in this process.

Nature of distress related to caste discrimination is both psychological and cultural, with an internalization of the gaze of upper castes and spatial-social dimensions within which both individual and institutional discrimination operates. Othering occurs from early stages in everyday social encounters which may be violent, normative, or transgressed. In ordinary social contexts, discrimination may be invisible as it is practised with deliberate attempts to stigmatize lower-caste people causing alienation and mental health problems in them. There are numerous instances of heinous crimes like getting stabbed for digging a well, deprived of water supply, murder of a person from Dalit community staged to look like suicide, being murdered for loving a person from upper caste, with the way people from Dalit community occasionally join political protests reminds us of the prejudice that remains a reality even today [B.B.C. News. Caste hatred in India. What it looks like, 7 May 2018].

In March 2016, a 22-year-old man was harassed to death for marrying a woman of a higher caste. His wife survived, and her father was sentenced to death.

Caste is not simply a law and order problem but a complex social problem of Indian society, causing immense suffering to the people from disadvantaged castes.

Buddhism Perspective

Buddhism is a psychology of the struggles of spirit and the experiences of the soul. It describes the four noble truths and that if there is suffering, it has a cause, and it can be suppressed following a proper path.

Life is considered a journey of suffering, and the processes of birth, death, and the separation from near and dear ones including cravings for unfulfilled desires are too painful.

Any kind of separation from our attachments is considered to be painful. All the great works including our dreams, hopes, our fears, and desires will be buried to become history at some point of time as nothing is permanent. Ignorance is the root cause through which our desire for false springs. Whatever things originate are also subject to destruction depending upon time variations. We can find that the continuity of an event is a product of succession of identities. Buddha cites the example of flame which maintains its unchanged appearance through every moment it is another not the same flame.

The law of universal causation, with its corollary of the eternal continuity of becoming, is the chief contribution of Buddhism.

Anything that comes into existence is impermanent which is conditioned by causes and conditions.

The order of universe is called *Niyama* or the process of going on, and the wheel of cosmic order exists without cause and effect relations. The true god is attainable only by the suppression of subjectivity of self and the development of universal consciousness. The development of uniting consciousness is the widening and expansion of our feelings for all.

Buddhist philosophy suggests eightfold path which can lead to cessation of suffering, but requires the development and exercise of wisdom and intellect, morality and adequate conduct, awareness, and meditation skills.

According to Buddhist psychology and the analysis of self-concepts, one's 'I' consciousness is constituted by five *Skandha* (aggregates) which includes

Rupa (physical form), *Vedana* (sensations and feelings), *Sonna* (perception), *Sankhara* (mental formations), and *Vimana* (consciousness).

Buddhism prescribes mindfulness as a technique where one tries to notice present thoughts, feelings, and sensations without judgement.

Mindfulness practice in a way is meant as a deterrent that purifies mind from sensual attachment to the body, a cleansing process whose final aim is a balanced attitude.

The Buddhist tradition talks about hindrances and awakening factors in the process of achieving mindfulness. The overcoming of hindrance factors such as sensual desires, restlessness, and ill-will is a pre-condition for the rise of awakening factors. Awakening is a process of achieving energy, joy, tranquility, concentration, and equanimity.

The practices of awakening can be achieved by different stages of breathing exercises by following four set of four steps comprising becoming are of the body, feelings, mind and dharmas. Mindfulness of breathing could be undertaken as a comprehensive meditation practice that proceeds through ways of establishing mindfulness.

For example there may be a situation for a teacher when

- his students do not listen to him;
- his students listen to him; and
- some listen, some do not listen.

According to Buddhist philosophy, the teacher should be neither happy nor unhappy in all three situations, and he should maintain equanimity remaining unaffected by repulsion or attraction.

Attitude of mindfulness is not governed by likes and dislikes and is free from desires or dejection in regard to the world. Plank refers to Christopher Germer (2005) in identifying three key concepts in therapeutic mindfulness: 1) Awareness 2) of the present experience 3) with acceptance (Plank, 2010).

Buddhist mindfulness emphasizes paying attention to the present moment, including the full spectrum of our experiences, the good, bad, and ugly to be at home in one's own skin. It is suggested that escape and avoidance are not solutions, and full enormity of life experiences should be embraced not resisted with a non-judging attitude, to be an impartial witness to the experience.

People should avoid judging thoughts and reactions to inner and outer experiences with a tendency to let go of thought and feelings that mind seems to hold on.

Therapeutic mindfulness is also considered as an awareness of the present moment with four cornerstones of observation, description, non-judgement, and participation (p. 22).

Meditation occupies a fundamental purpose of developing a realization of fundamental conditions with insight (*Vipassana*). Theravada scripture *Visuddhimagga* differs between two main kinds of meditation orientation:

concentration (*Samatha*) and insight (*Vipassana*). According to Buddhist philosophy, the purpose of Vipassana is to provide realizations or insight about fundamental conditions of existence, an experience-based understanding of how existence is in continuous change (*anicca*), how this instability has no permanence (*anatta*), and how this results in disenchantment (*dukha*).

The term satic (right mindfulness) is an important aspect of developing *bodhi* (awakening) and the final liberation (*Nirvana*).

Wisdom

According to Buddhism, wisdom refers to the gradual development of insight that allows and facilitates an individual to recover from ontological addiction of deep-rooted belief in 'I' or self and impaired functionality arising from such beliefs.

Loving Kindness and Compassion

Buddhist construal of loving kindness and compassion does not involve pity, and it is described with four immeasurable attitudes of (i) joy, (ii) loving kindness, (iii) compassion, and (iv) equanimity. Loving kindness is a fundamental orientation for welfare of all, and compassion refers to the wish for all beings to be free from suffering and its causes.

Equanimity is considered as an attitude of unconditional and impartial cultivation of loving kindness and compassion for all. Each of these conduct-related practices of joy, equanimity compassion, or patience should be conducted unconditionally of either–or approach. Talking about patience, an Indian Buddhist saint of eighth century Santideva (1997) stated that 'the mind does not find peace nor does it enjoy pleasure and joy nor does it find sleep or fortitude when the thorn of hatred dwells in the heart' (p. 60). According to Buddhism, patience leads to connectedness which is a state beyond all hope and fear and beyond any desire to modify the present moment.

Emptiness

Buddhist philosophy of emptiness asserts that all phenomena including the self are empty of intrinsic existence. Buddhism emptiness theory implies that there is no logical or scientific plausibility of the principles on which an individual constructs their self-concept, and the notion of inherent existence is fundamentally flawed. Emptiness (Pali Sunnata and Sanskrit Sunyata) refers to the idea from Buddhist teaching that emptiness is a way of life which suggests that phenomena including self are devoid of intrinsic existence, implying a concept of non-self. From the Mahayana perspective, emptiness is viewed through the lens of interconnectedness, middle path, and *Yogacar* that all phenomena are dream like.

All the phenomena are interconnected in nature, and their origin is dependent on each other.

For example a flower manifests its dependence on water, soil, air, gardener, and many insects that died to produce nutrients for the soil. Therefore, a flower does not exist in isolation, but it is with various interconnected elements, and it is empty of inherently existing self. Similarly, *Yogacar* position demonstrates that the waking-state reality has properties similar to a dream-like state which seems contradictory to existing beliefs. But, in reality, there are no actual grounds on which to distinguish between the ultimate nature of how phenomena exist in dreaming and waking reality. In the contemporary psychology, ideas of self-worth and self-image are constructed as the explicit acceptance of a discrete 'self' entity. The emphasis on majority of the perspectives in psychology sense of self is considered to be distinct from others, and a desire to protect the self is considered to be a fundamental objective.

Non-attachment to self can foster an increase of spiritual awareness and affection towards others.

A closely related principle of emptiness is the concept of impermanence which means all phenomena will cease to be, which keeps changing every moment, and it can't be located in time and space. An acceptance of the view of the impermanent nature of existence may help in the recovery of the grieving process. Emptiness theory asserts that when mind stops being attached to certain phenomena (including itself), it lets go of the idea of existing as a discrete self-entity and it expands to its full capacity. The capacity of mind expanding to its full range can be understood with the analogy of a wave in the ocean. Although wave emerges as a discrete identity, but in no time it is separate from the ocean. A deceptive mind may be compared to a wave which only sees itself as a wave, but a mind realizing its full capacity may be considered to a wave that acts as an expression of ocean. Even scientific theories appear to be gradually adding credence to the idea that phenomena are empty of intrinsic existence.

The *Bhagavad Gita* Perspective

The *Bhagavad Gita* is one of the finest lessons of philosophy, religion, and ethics. The struggling of human life passes through several dark and bright phases, and teachings of Gita suggest the path for enlightenment.

The philosophical systems of Gita are not merely metaphysical but enduring truths of spiritual experience and verifiable facts of psychological possibilities woven into perfect harmony. The language and thought of the *Gita* avoid rigid determination, and it embraces spiritual truth and the doctrine of practicality.

The *Gita* is a rich source and synthesis of a discipline in the preparation for renouncement through multiple paths.

The *Gita* prescribes a perfect balance between one's actions and spiritual realization and above all selfless performance of duties. It is often possible to experience a clash of interests occurring in performing our duties, and it can be solved through the idea of *Kartavyam Karma* (the work that is to be done) without any expectation of the fruits of action. The *Gita* teaches a method which is within the reach of all struggling individuals who are faced with terrible sufferings to find the way for illumination.

Lord Krishna, the very god, like a teacher addresses Arjuna during the time of his crisis and stands for the infinite into the finite, the God in man concealed within the folds of flesh and the powers of sense. The *Gita* argues that the soul is free from cravings, attachments, and egoism of 'I-ness' and 'myness'. Ignorance is considered as main cause of pain and suffering in the pursuance of human goals. Attachment to emotions and sensations causes grief and sorrow, and people should not grieve for death as birth and death are like cycles of the immortal soul.

The equality of divine consciousness depends upon a perfect equality in the soul, mind, and heart to realize our true sense of oneness.

Yoga is a method for transformation and attaining a spiritual condition of universal equality.

Samadhi is the highest state of bliss when a person loses consciousness of objects, surrounding, and desire by reaching an inner state of freedom, free from attractions and repulsions. It is very difficult to get rid of our senses, and it is not possible to do so with intelligence or will, rather taking refuge in the divine through yoga is the solution.

The peace of a person is affected by outward emotions, longings, impulsions, and passions which lead to loss in the power of calm and mastery.

The *Gita* favours action over knowledge and intelligence, and it further emphasizes *Niskama Karma* (desireless action) as the superior form of action.

One's ego and sense can be overcome through completeness of works in the knowledge of the divine. The major sources of our suffering comes from our enslavement to appearances, and our giving in to the dualities of good and evil, grief and joy following the world of maya.

The perception of assumptions and ignorance of self-identification is bewildered by the ego sense. The self-assertions of ego sense are the broken and distorted shadows in our minds of external self, but the self within is free from limitations of consequences.

There is a need to understand the distinction between suppression (*Nirgraha*) and self-control (*Samyama*). The former is a violence done to the nature by will which results into depression, and the latter is the control of lower self by the light of higher self which provides those powers, their right action, and their maximum efficiency: *Yogah Karmasu Kausalam.*

In a particular state, people keep on desiring but do not get satisfied with it, and in a different stage people neither desire nor crave for the satisfactions arising from desires. People have this common illusion of desires and have the impression that their desires are born within. In reality, desires are imported like waves from others, and a tendency for possessiveness of desires may look like a natural desire, which is a false impression.

In reality, the desires of lower impulses like jealousy or envy, hatred or violence are external waves which overwhelm and invade a person, which is not an intrinsic part of nature. The desires of lower impulses have no character or personality – they manifest in the same way whoever provides a space for it. When the psychic organization of a person allows the lust for control, domination and weaknesses of love and hate bring panics, and fear imposes feelings of grief.

In order to get rid of suffering, one should attempt to get rid of desire being manifested through someone, and a refusal to accept those desires for manifestation will tire the desires, which will leave one quietly.

Dharma in the *Bhagavad Gita* is not a mere creed, but it is a way and law of self moulding by which one can grow towards divinity. Avatarhood is an extraordinary manifestation of divine qualities within the common man. The concept of avatarhood in the *Gita* is a dual phenomenon of divinity and humanity in which humanity can acquire divinity enabled by grand modification of consciousness. The world is like a theatre in which the struggle between inner and outer powers goes on, and *Dharma* comes to aid to overcome outer struggles.

Our attitude towards life and ability to witness wonderful at every moment lifts us towards calm and virtuous pathways. The divine workers do not claim for the doership, abandoning all attachments to the fruits of their works. The liberated person does everything with no personal hopes without making no turbulent response to the touches of outward things. All human souls are capable of acquiring spiritual personality of working and are free from egoistic reactions, which offer a perfect equality in the soul and the nature. One of the key characteristics of the philosophy of *Gita* is its emphasis upon transcendent Godhead who is present everywhere. Yoga is a method for dedicating our entire existence to the supreme through higher levels of consciousness.

The secret of Godhead is not mystical rather cosmic divinity, and individual divinity is connected to the same spectrum. The synthesis of knowledge, work, and devotion can bring awakening to the identity of eternal delight and oneness. The profitless circling of ego, hunting after finite things, and earthly hunger of the intellect body and senses are devoid of true consciousness.

It is a tendency of blind hope that chases after transient but misses the eternal, and this may cause suffering.

The divine comes alive through an attitude of detachment, and through *sadhana* even a person of evil conduct can turn into a saint. In the spiritual life, all man-made distinctions cease before the divine light and the wide omnipotence of an impartial power.

When the knowledge of the field and its knower is united, it acquires the capacity of a divine teacher.

Three equalities of *Sattva*, *Rajas*, and *Tamas* produce a vital effect on human beings and are inextricably intertwined in all cosmic existence. *Tamas* as nature's power of nescience is the principle of inertia is strongest in material nature. Whatever is predominantly governed by Tamas, tends in its force to a sluggish action and immobility, driving a person in mechanical round of energy. The principle of *Rajas* as the power of active seeking, enlightened by desire, has its hold on vital nature. Therefore, *Rajas* always turns a person to action and desire, but struggles carried out to achieve success are marred by the after-taste of insufficiency, disappointment, and suffering. *Sattva* as the power of possessing and harmonizing knowledge has its strongest hold in the intelligence and the will of the person. *Rajas* is a state of assimilation, equilibrium, and harmony, which brings happiness, mastery, and security in the person.

In all persons, there is a higher or lower proportions of a mingling of the *gunas* and a predominance of one or the other *guna*.

Yoga of supreme person known as *Purushottama* provides escape from ego and, united with the divine soul, lives purified and liberated. Ignorance means *Avidya* separated from truth brings falsehood and sufferings. *Askesis* practised with a supreme faith of serenity with no desire or fruit is considered to be sattvic.

Askesis which is freely formed for the source of gaining respect and honour is the characteristic of *Rajasic*. The *Askesis* done with a view to hurt to the feelings of others is guided by *tamasic* tendency.

The best *Dana* (gift) is given for the sake of giving to one from whom no benefit is expected in return, which is known as *atmadan* or *atma-samarpan,* and it is considered as highest form of *Sattvic Dana*.

In the formula of Om, Tat, and Sat considered as creator of the Brahmans, the vedas and sacrifices in which Tat indicates the absolute, sat indicates the supreme and OM is the symbol of the triple Brahman; the outward looking, the inward or subtle and the superconscient causal purusha. Each letter A, U, and M indicates one of these three in the ascending order, and the syllable as a whole brings out the fourth state, Turiya, which rises to the absolute.

The *Gita* while describing the concept of sacrifice (Tyaga) suggests action with a renunciation of desire and not a flight to the monastery, the cave, or the hill-top.

Following one's own nature (*Swabhava*) is a better way for obtaining self-control, purity, and spiritual truth. Lack of self-discipline is a source of myriads of sufferings, and self-discipline (*Sadhana*) breaks down limitations into opportunities. By the term Brahman, the *Gita* intends the immutable self-existence which is the highest self-expression of the Divine on whose unalterable eternity all the rest, all that moves and evolves are found. By *Adhyatma,* it means *Swabhava*, the spiritual way, and law of being of the soul in the supreme nature.

The *Bhagavad Gita* in brief suggests the path of Karma, and without expectations of desires people can derive joy and happiness in their work, which is normally a great source of suffering for most of the people.

Karma, Bhakti, and Gyan Marg

The philosophy of the *Gita* prescribes divine actions and sacrifice of knowledge by turning the mind towards the divine. It also suggests enlargement of our mental consciousness free from egoistic dualities. The dialogue and relationship between inner awareness and outer action are the key theme in the *Bhagavad Gita*. Arjuna's possibility of killing his own relatives poses a great moral dilemma which is explained by Lord Krishna, through *Dharma* or carrying out moral duty in the context of a situation. True Karmayoga means that we should act with such awareness that no attachment or act expectations are aligned with it.

The conduct of righteousness suppressing all selfishness is the true path of a Karmayogi. Even if people fail in their efforts, good actions can help them advance towards completeness. The spirit of doing good for others can be achieved through the ideals of *Loksangrah* or the solidarity of the world. The hesitant Arjuna was persuaded by Krishna to fight, not for the attraction of glory or lust of the kingdom, but for protecting the law of righteousness. All good work should be performed with the purity of mind, which leads one to wisdom. Karma performed as a sacrifice to the God is considered to be superior and effective. The Karma theory of the *Gita* also empowers individuals, and Karma is considered only a condition and not a destiny. Many of our sufferings are born out of idleness, and following the path of action can improve the mental health to positivity and wellness.

Bhakti

The *Bhakti Marg*, or the path of devotion, indicates emotional attachment which is distinct from knowledge or action. The sacrifice and faith of love through emotional route lead to the perception of the supreme. The love of an object is falsehood, contributing to the element of separateness. The sacrifice of love to the divine transcends to a higher state and gates of spirit be open for them. The *Gita* always emphasizes that God is present in each individual, and prospects of a harmonious union with God depends upon a vision of delight.

People who completely devote themselves to the love of God experience happiness (*priti*), and those who remain in the absence of God experience sadness (*viraha*). The process of undivided devotion to the supreme makes one free from misery and filled with joy and peace.

Faith is a vital element of the *Bhakti Marg*, and some forms of worship done with devotion are helpful for purifying the heart and mind to get higher consciousness.

There are people who involve in discussion in vain, but the highest form of *Bhakti* is continuity (*nirantarta*) with intense love for God.

The process of devotion turns into truth of the oneness with God in the universe known as *Vasudevah Sarvam Iti.*

True devotion is an unselfish act in which a devotee is immersed in an embracing beneficent love that does not expect any return.

The true conduct of a devotee lies in his absolute self-surrender and the complete dedication to the God.

Part time devotions and selfish motives can become the source of one's miseries. *Bhakti Marg* is considered to be a powerful route to well-being.

Jnana Marg

All knowledge forms are an awakening to identity when the inner being is touched by the light and complete commitment to the God-head towards perfect realization. The knowledge turns into an adoration of the *Purushottama.* It is a universal pursuit of infinite in the finite, a vision and embracing the one in his oneness. The divine seekers of knowledge for the divine themselves become the inhabitants of divinity. The divine thinker himself becomes the enlightened one through offerings towards Godhead in his nature and being. It would be apt to mention one of the verses of *Bhagavad Gita* which mentions:

> I am the supreme path and goal, the sustainer, the master, the witness, the abode and the refuge, well-wisher seeking no return. Origin and end, the foundation and resting place to which all beings return at the time of universal destructions and the enduring seed of all.
>
> (Chapters 9–18, Verse18]

The knowledge of the Godhead can be acquired by all the wise or unwise through destruction of apparent contradiction and finding their vision with the master.

The process of seeing the Divine is a condition of conscious self-surrender and enlarge itself into a greater Seeking to the Supreme Purushottama.

There are several ways people follow to approach the divinity, and some of it may involve physical/material acts (such as decorating an idol). Others may involve mental consecration or symbolic gesture to the symbol, and finally these acts and symbol make oneself fit to unite with the divinity. It is very rare occasion when people combine all these, which becomes a deterrent in seeking oneness. The knowledge principle applied in the *Gita* is that of developing inner surrender and having trust and confidence in the divine.

All kinds of sorrow and grief will disappear in the bliss of all-blissful, and human error and sin are transformed into strength, truth, and purity of the eternal.

The inner vision (*drishti*) is a powerful mechanism through which things unseen also become evident. What hides the truth from our vision is not merely the fault of the intellect, but also the passion of selfishness. In order to kindle vision, the fire of passion and the tumult of desire must be suppressed. The knowledge perspective of the *Gita* carries us beyond one-sided conclusion, and narrow viewpoints to the comprehensive truth and eternal spirit lead to the most complete experience. To achieve this eternal calm, two ways of yoga and *jnana* are suggested in which yoga indicates the suppression of mental activity (*vriti-nirodha*), and *jnana* is true comprehension (*samyagaveksanam*).

The *Gita* does not put excess emphasis on yoga and suggests the control of senses and indifference to attractions through the growth of knowledge.

Critical Evaluation

Modern life system is characterized by fear, anxiety, competition, envy with long working hours, lack of work–life balance, and hunger for success leading to the amplification of one's ego. Consider the life of a man in the city. They are continuously in the grip of a mechanized lifestyle with hardly any scope for escape. These people may have a charming house, good family, and children. The typical routine of an urbanite with exceptions is guided in the manner that he wakes up in the morning for his office work, dictates or is dictated by the office work, talks on phone and mails several people, comes home in the late evening, readies for dinner, and sleeps. Year by year, he grows more lonely, his attention grows more concentrated, and life outside office and professional domain has least meaning. The official religion and glory demand that he/she should be busy, and mind is persuaded that it is his/her duty to pursue success by being busy and it all makes him/her too anxious to be happy.

Genuine irrational fear of consequences of losing the status enters into anxieties of a professional person. Sometimes, childhood fears of poverty haunt in later stages with excess emphasis on money as an extraordinary factor of wellness.

Material success is seen as a mark of success at the cost of fundamental avenues of happiness.

Unless a person has been aware of what is to do with success, the achievement of it inevitably leaves him/her a prey of boredom.

The suffering arises from believing in the false notion of life according to which life is a contest, a competition of ego battle for status achievement, in which respect is to be accorded to the victor.

It is not only the work that is poisoned by the philosophy of competition, even leisure is poisoned as much.

The prolonged periods of competition and ego conflicts produce nervous fatigue, various psychological processes of escape, and the disappearance of positivity in the end.

The machine age has been heavily structured into societies and has tremendously affected all aspects of people's life and, most notably, mass alienation. Technologies continue to play a great role in the achievements of nations.

Social theory of technology and alienation described from the lens of dialectical materialism propose social tension and conflict, causing suffering to the masses.

Human struggle and competition result in differences in the distribution of income, power, and control between those who control the means of production and those who are at the receiving end.

Many theorists viewed technology itself as constituting a realm of the sublime that is revolutionizing art, everyday life and human subjectivity providing higher dimensions to human experience.

Critics from the philosophical community hold technology responsible for humans losing touch with bodies, nature, and other people with focal things and practices leading to alienation and dehumanization. Clifford Stoll's Silicon snake oil. Second thoughts on information highways (1995) provide a technophobic epistle, which provides a fascinating contrast with Bill Gates' *The Road Ahead* (1995) contradicting everything that Gate affirms.

Extreme post-modern technophobic critiques are found in Arthur Kroker and Michael Weinstein who in their book *Data Trash* (1995) suggest that contemporary culture has crashed, imploded into hyper-reality and that people have lost touch with reality altogether, being ruled by a new virtual class.

Technology has acquired the shape of religion for many, but critical side of it also highlights several social anxieties leading to psychological suffering. From a Marxist critique, perspective labour under capitalism was alienated because one was estranged from one's potential of creativity and self-realization as a many-sided being as people are forced to engage in specialized and one-sided labour.

The painful aspects of socially lived experiences have psychological implications.

Social suffering is produced by inequalities in the society and practices against the marginalized groups. In the Indian context, many cases related to caste atrocities and poverty prejudices lead to discrimination and social suffering.

Violence against women is a deep-rooted social problem of Indian society.

Acts of gender-based violence results in life-long suffering which may include physical aggression, sexual coercion, or controlling behaviours.

Perpetrators of violence against women are people from the same society, and its causes are associated with social and cultural attitude, stereotypes, unequal gender, power patriarchy, and two factors harming the well-being of women. Such problems are man-made, and a long-term planning aimed at eradicating the violence against women should be undertaken and implemented on the evidence-based realities. The prevalence of crime against women varies from culture to culture, hence strengthening the attitude of equality from an interdisciplinary perspective can help to reduce the suffering.

The biomedical model of providing remedy from suffering focuses more upon client–therapist relations, but in reality it is highly influenced by sociocultural factors. Lifestyle problems do not have merely physiological origin, but in majority of the situations, family, society, and larger issues of the surrounding environment do play a crucial role in its higher or lower rates of prevalence of psychological problems.

Several spiritual dimensions and perspectives do play a significant role in the suffering and healing mechanisms. Spiritual beliefs can tremendously support the healing process. The practice of meditation and yoga has been found to be very effective in the process of healing. Strong scientific evidence suggests that individuals who regularly participle in spiritual worship or prayers and related activities are healthier and possess greater healing capabilities.

Spirituality and health is a less explored domain by the healthcare professionals. Indigenous cultures hold no separation between healing and a connection to the sacred. It is very clear that mind, body, and heart act in collaboration, and spiritual practices focus on striking a harmonious balance between the three. The mind and heart are important sources contributing to the physical symptoms. The philosophy of Buddhism and the *Bhagavad Gita* provide an in-depth understanding of the causes of suffering and ways to enlightenment. The practice of the Medicine Buddha, the supreme healer (*Sangye Menla* in Tibetan), is a powerful method for healing oneself and others. The concepts related to the truth of human suffering and the truth of cessation and suffering are very well explained in the Buddhist teachings.

Buddhism prescribes the practical rather than theoretical ways to attain wisdom and understanding of the self. Buddhist approach suggests logical tenets and then provides a way of personally experiencing them through self-reflection. For example the basic teachings of four noble truths observe that everything is impermanent, including one's own life, and the impermanence of the materialistic world is a primary cause of suffering. Buddhist teachings attempt to help humans to cure themselves not by changing others but by changing themselves.

The treatment of suffering in Buddhism is divided into virtue (*Sila*), concentration (*Samadhi*), and cognition (*Panna*) Understood as behavioural treatment, mental treatment, and cognitive treatment, respectively.

Mindfulness-based therapies share common aims with Buddhist psychology. The concepts of loving kindness, gratitude, and compassion are extremely relevant for the purpose of healing which finds detailed expression in Buddhist teachings.

Buddhism notion of selflessness and reduced attachment to ego or self enable individuals to be free from misery. Many of our problems stem from conditioned identity and ignorance which are considered the roots of neurosis. The delusion of self exists as a result of one's way of thinking and behaviour. One of the aims of Buddhist teachings is to enable an individual to see the reality of self-nature through self-investigating his/her personal relationship with others. The guiding principles of confession and reflection, compassion and consciousness of body and mind can bring far-reaching positive changes in one's behaviour.

Modern society is too complicated with the complexities of domination of one religious identity over the other, powerful nation subjugating the rights of undeveloped countries, rich suppressing the poor, the educated and powerful dominating over the resources in an inequal manner, and the goals of equitable development of humans and humanity seeming to be an illusion. The modern concepts of scientific intervention do bring some changes in improving some sectors, but new challenges and frontiers of discontent start posing fresh challenges.

A paradigm shift in thinking and orientation towards the concept of human progress and development is the need of the time. Treating individuals from the perspective of individual-centric frame of reference may not be able to bring wholesome changes in the direction of ideal human development. Buddhism as a philosophy and practice can solve many of the problems of conflict and violence that humanity as a whole is facing, and isolated treatment method can't be a proper solution to the problems we are confronting in the contemporary society.

The teachings of the *Bhagavad Gita* suggest that causes of our suffering are related to desires, expectations, and claim of doership for our actions. The ambivalence between duties and being judgmental makes us worried about the outcomes. Majority of fears and conflicts of human mind originate due to the tendency to appropriate the infinite of reality into finite of parochial objectives expressed as I, me, or mine. The issues of guilt, fear of failure, and anger are important emotions aggravating our suffering, and the *Gita*'s teachings suggest that conquering the urge of our egos can lead us to the path of healing. The concept of equanimity or importance of equal-mindedness has been repeatedly emphasized in various verses of the *Gita*.

It is suggested in the *Gita* to maintain balance in pleasure and pain, and this type of patience makes one eligible for eternal life. The worldly pleasure is finite in nature, but at some points of time whether it is material or any other type of power. *Gita* teachings reiterate that one should do his duty without any bondage to the attachment of its fruits, and they should be equipoised both in success and failure. The state of perfect equanimity is the state of blessedness in which one establishes his/her unity with the divine (*Purushottama*).

Everything in nature displays three qualities (*guna*): the *Sattva*, *Rajas,* and *Tamas* representing spiritual goodness, passion and desires, and darkness, respectively. All three *gunas* are present in a person with the domination of one over the others. The lowest order of *Gunas* is represented through *Tamas* which makes a person aggressive and violent. The next order of

Guna is represented by *Rajas* which makes a person take pleasure in name and fame. The highest order of *Guna* is *Sattva* in which a person sacrifices the ego or personal interest for the larger interest of society.

People through awareness and yoga can transform from lower *gunas* of *Tamas* to higher *Guna* of *Sattva* and through engaging in virtuous actions.

Sattva is considered to be illuminating, and people influenced by it lean towards purity, knowledge, peacefulness, and happiness.

The theory of *Nishkama Karma* has great importance, and it suggests doing action without being dependent on its outcomes.

Reflections from *Swadharma* (one's own self) and less importance to the rituals are considered helpful in the process of overcoming grief. The *Gita* is an excellent philosophy and a practical guide par excellence whose principles can be applied in the healing process of everyday problems in the society.

Summary

Suffering is a state of distress which threatens the well-being of a person. The concept of suffering has several dimensions which can be physical, social, or psychological. When an individual feels disconnected and alienated and experiences stress due to a lack of integrity and sense of coherence, this stage maybe described as the stage of suffering. The concept of suffering indicates a loss of one's sense of worth or meaning.

The perception of suffering brings a sense of weakness and vulnerability to the person, which poses a threat to the well-being of that person. The concept of suffering has been explained with the help of sacred scriptures like the *Gita* and many other mythological texts.

Social suffering is a result of historical, cultural, and social practices of inequality between people on the bases of caste, religion, ethic intensity, economic status, and gender. Inequality is a problem in itself, and it is closely related to social sufferings of the marginal. Inequality undermines social justice, and the interconnectedness of different kinds of inequalities means some groups have consistently worse opportunities and life conditions than those of their fellow citizens. People face discrimination on the bases of caste, gender, and economic status, which is guided by stigma and social stereotypes, undermining their social participation and opportunities for healthy living. Prejudice and negative stereotypes result in violence against women and the poor. Inequality also increases the vulnerability of societies and of particular marginal groups.

Charmaz (2002) talked about the concept of silenced suffering. Culturally authorized meanings and interpretation play important roles in the coherence and perception of suffering. In the Indian context, the case of social suffering related to caste, poverty, and gender status is very much prevalent.

Buddhism identifies the origin of suffering in the ignorance and craving for pleasures. Suffering is considered to be the creation of an individual, and it can cease to exist when the impermanent nature of the world is recognized. Suffering can also be alleviated through mindfulness and concentration. Meditation is the vehicle for enlightenment. Buddhist teachings describe three main types of sufferings. The first is called 'the suffering of suffering', the second 'the suffering of change', and the third 'the suffering of conditioning'. According to Buddhism, five aggregates of matter, sensations, perceptions, mental formations, and consciousness contribute to *Dukha* (suffering). The noble eightfold path leads to the elimination of the personality and self which contributes to non-self and a path to *Nirvana* (salvation).

Buddhism also suggests that *Dukha* (suffering) is an innate characteristic of the world, and it is caused because of craving, desire, or attachment; cessation of *Dukha* can be attained by renouncement, and finally eightfold path is suggested to lead to the renouncement of desire and cessation of *Dukha*.

The concept of liberating insight is considered important for enlightenment.

Many of the illusions and sufferings of human being can be controlled and calmed following principles of Buddhism. Psychiatrists, scientists, doctors and psychologists use the practice of Buddhist teachings for healing mental problems of their clients.

The philosophy of the *Bhagavad Gita* can be used to overcome the sufferings of the people in this materialistic age. According to it, *atman* (soul) can't be slain and described as eternal while physical body is considered to be transient. The *Gita* emphasizes doing our Karma, renouncing the attachment for doership, and people should follow *Swadharma* and discharge their duties.

The teachings of the *Gita* again and again emphasize that one should cultivate an attitude of non-attachment, and an individual should live in the world like water on a lotus leaf. The *Gita* formulates theory of three paths of Janan yoga for a person of wisdom and rational temperament, Bhakti yoga for devotion and emotional temperament, and Karma yoga for a person of action, and these paths are not in conflict with each other. The central teaching of the Gita is the attainment of the final beautiful perfection of life or eternal freedom.

The actual aim of life is a complete identification with the divine, which exists in the past, present, and future; which does not have a beginning, middle, or end; which has neither parts nor limbs; and which is neither subtle nor gross.

The problem of likes and dislikes can be controlled through *Sadhana*. Every human is affected by three *gunas* of *Sattwa*, *Rajas*, and *Tamas*.

It is possible for humans to transform the lower qualities of *Tamas* to *Rajas* and *Sattva* through action. It is a philosophy to dispel the darkness of suffering through the light of embodied self which is eternal. The self is considered to be indestructible and infinite; and sword can't cut it, fire cannot burn it, and wind cannot dry it. People must not grieve for material losses of any kind; even death should not be mourned as the physical body perceived to be a combination of the five elements return to their source.

Fighting for a righteous cause is considered a part of one's duty. Performing actions with equanimity or the doctrine of point in action is considered as superior form of action.

Purification of heart through Karma yoga leads to fearlessness.

The delusion of me, mine, and I is the source of one's misery, and a person free from attraction and repulsion attains peace and happiness.

The wandering senses push people towards miseries, but one can attain peace by abandoning desires and longings without the sense of mine and egoism.

So many types of doubts arising due to *Moha* (attachment) become the source of delusion, and this can be transformed into perfection by doing all actions as a divine offering, imbued with a spirit of non-attachment and sacrifice.

The right attitude of detachment from desires leads to divine glory of peace, bliss, and freedom. The teachings of the *Bhagavad Gita* can be a great source of healing to overcome the pleasures and pain, becoming obstacles in life.

The ego problems in our relationships of me, mine, and I can be controlled by following *Sattvic Guna*.

Suffering and healing should be dealt with multi-perspective approach as their meaning and impact vary along different perspectives. There are types and stages of suffering, and they should not be construed with the notion of all or none perspective. The feelings of pain and suffering also have positive connotations from spiritual points of view. There are sufferings, which lead to new identity and innovations. Spiritual ideas often produce tremendous amount of optimism and hope from meaninglessness to meaningfulness and purpose of human existence. Contemporary medical models of empirical evidence approach treat illnesses on the basis of anatomical, physiological, and biochemical terms. Physicians' and clinicians' attitude of treating patients and their illnesses from the biomedical perspective lacks other important components of compassion, empathy, and altered states of consciousness. In other words, majority of clinicians treat clients' problems and clients as capable human beings in an isolated and compartmentalized manner. It is important to explore the multi-perspective and discover the moral/spiritual foundations of the clients. Compassion, empathy, mindfulness, and attitude of equanimity cultivated through yoga and meditation can offer great support to recover from suffering by performing concrete healing actions. If the objective conditions of a client are analysed to alleviate the suffering of individuals, the role of subjective components of spiritual understanding can facilitate deep hope in the healing process.

Much disharmony caused to a person can be negated and harmony regained by transforming the conditioned thinking to insightful and reflective understanding. The perspectives of Buddhism and the *Bhagavad Gita* can certainly provide a strong support in understanding and resolution of the suffering and healing processes. So many problems that people in contemporary society face these days are based upon superficial ego problems and lack of discipline with the lifestyle. These scriptures provide a meaningful support for leading a life free from ego conflicts and based upon peace, tranquility, and integration of the mind, body. and soul in a blissful way with connectedness to the nature and divinity. Lifestyle changes followed in a disciplined manner and mindful ways of achieving happiness can solve a variety of problems the people of modern age are experiencing. No one-day theory can bring magical results in terms of wellness, and lives have to be lived as a process of accepting the reality and finding ways to move ahead with the eternal calm. Suffering and healing are not independent of each other, hence treating them in a mindful way will be considered a pragmatic approach to move in the journey of life.

Think Box

Compare and contrast the Indian and Western notions of suffering and healing.

Key Points:

- Suffering and healing are not limited to physiological symptoms, and they are also influenced a lot by moral and spiritual meanings.
- The insightful moments and meaning that come through the sacrifice of suffering can lead to self-transcendence.
- The person-centred dogma derived from social institutions medicine confine sickness or suffering located in the biological symptoms.
- Collective suffering of the people is labelled as social pathology, and its solutions are social and political in nature.
- Stigma and discrimination affect people being internalized by them, which has silencing effects on them, preventing and seeking support.
- Violence against women by their partners and sexual violence can negatively affect women's physical and mental health.
- Caste identity also influences individuals' self-concept, and it has implications for a self-esteem and psychological coherence.
- Buddhism is a psychology of the struggles of spirit and the experiences of the soul.
- Buddhism prescribes mindfulness as a technique where one tries to notice present thoughts, feelings, and sensations without judgement.
- Non-attachment to self can foster an increase of spiritual awareness and affection towards others.

Key Terms:

Buddhism, Suffering, Healing, Self-transcendence, Popularizational, Caste-discrimination, Suffering, Untouchability, Mindfulness, Wisdom

References

Beteille, A. (2011). *The Andre Betteille omnibus*. Oxford university Press.

Bourdieu, P. et al. (1999). *The weight of the world: Social suffering in contemporary society* (P. P. Ferguson, Trans.). Polity Press.

Cassell, E. J. (2004). *The nature of suffering and the goals of medicine* (2nd ed.). Oxford University Press.

Charmaz, K. (2002). Stories and silences: Disclosures and self in chronic illness. *Qualitative Inquiry, 8*, 302–328.

Deshpande, A. (2011). *The grammar of caste: Economic discrimination in contemporary India*. Oxford University Press.

Gergen, K. J. (1994). *Realities and relationships soundings in social construction*. Harvard University Press.

Germer, C. K. (2005). Mindfulness: What it is? What does it matter? In C. K. Germer, R. S. Siegel, & P. R. Falton (Eds.), *Mindfulness and psychotherapy* (pp. 3–27). The Guildford Press.

Gorringe, H., & Rafanell, I. (2007). The embodiment of caste: Oppression, protest and change. *Sociology, 41*(1), 97–114.

Klienman, A. (1998). *The illness narratives: Suffering healing and human condition*. Basic Books.

Kroker, A., & Weinstein, M. A. (1995). *Data trash: The theory of the virtual class*. New World Perspectives.

Lewis-Fernández, R., & Kleinman, A. (1994). Culture, personality, and psychopathology. *Journal of Abnormal Psychology, 103*(1), 67–71.

Marsella, A. J. (1998). Toward a "global community psychology" meeting the needs of a changing world. *American Psychologist, 53*, 1282–1291.

Morris, D. B. (1991). *The culture of pain*. University of California Press.

Morris, D. B. (1998). *Illness and culture in the postmodern age*. University of California Press.

Plank, K. (2010). Mindful medicine: The growing trend of mindfulness-based therapies in the Swedish health care system. *Finnish Journal of Ethnicity & Migration, 5*(2), 47–55.

Santideva, A. (1997). *A guide to Bodhisattva way of life* (V. A. Wallace & B. A. Wallace, Trans.). Snow Lion.

Turner, J. C., Hogg, M. A., Oakes, P. J., Reicher, S. D., & Wetherell, M. S. (1987). *Rediscovering the social group: A self-categorization theory*. Blackwell.

United Nations (1993). *Declaration on the elimination of violence against women* UN.

Wallace, V. A., & Wallace, B. A. (1997). *A guide to the bodhisattva way of life by Santideva*. TBI Publishers. ISBN: 978-1569570494.

Index

For Product Safety Concerns and Information please contact our EU representative GPSR@taylorandfrancis.com Taylor & Francis Verlag GmbH, Kaufingerstraße 24, 80331 München, Germany